The Beginner's Guide to Medicinal Plants

The Beginner's Guide to Medicinal Plants

50 Essential Wild Herbs to Identify, Harvest, and Use

AMBER ROBINSON, PhD

ROCKRIDGE
PRESS

I dedicate this book to my grandma
Doris, who has been using medicinal
and edible plants her whole life, and
who passed this passion on to me!

Copyright © 2023 by Rockridge Press

All rights reserved. No part of this publication may be reproduced, stored in a retrieval system, or transmitted in any form or by any means, electronic, mechanical, photocopying, recording, scanning, or otherwise, without the prior written permission of the Publisher. Requests to the Publisher for permission should be addressed to the Permissions Department, Rockridge Press, 1955 Broadway, Suite 400, Oakland, CA 94612.

First Rockridge Press trade paperback edition 2023

Rockridge Press and the Rockridge Press logo are trademarks or registered trademarks of Callisto Media Inc. and/or its affiliates in the United States and other countries and may not be used without written permission.

For general information on our other products and services, please contact our Customer Care Department within the United States at (866) 744-2665, or outside the United States at (510) 253-0500.

Paperback ISBN: 979-8-88650-826-0 | eBook ISBN: 979-8-88650-830-7

Manufactured in the United States of America

Interior and Cover Designer:
Brieanna H. Felschow & Helen Bruno
Art Producer: Melissa Malinowksy & Stacey Stambaugh
Editor: Laura Cerrone
Production Editor: Rachel Taenzler
Production Manager: Riley Hoffman

Photographs and Illustrations by Shutterstock: © Sodel Vladyslav: front cover, ii, 51; Dionis-vera: front cover, ii, 81, 99; © spline_x: front cover, ii, 45, 53, 71, 117; © Anton Starikov: front cover, ii, 43, 101; © Madlen: front cover, ii, 55, 111; © Kalcutta: front cover, ii, 131; © Yevheniia Lytvynovych: front cover (tools); © Anna Paff: iii, throughout; © krolya25: 2; © C Teubner: 14; © nika-lit: 26; © Valentyn Volkov: 47; © domnitsky: 49, 91; © azure1: 57; © jopelka: 59; © Scisetti Alfio: 61, 123, 125, 139, back cover; © Emilio100: 65, back cover; © Diana Taliun: 73; © Snowbelle: 77; © Yuriy Chertok: 79, back cover; © OSINSKIH AGENCY: 83, back cover; © Manfred Ruckszio: 87, 121; © Ilizia: 89; © Hortimages: 95; © Marty Kropp: 97; © Zadiraka Evgenii: 103; © Fishman64: 109; © Superheang168: 113; © Peter Milto: 127; © Volosina: 129; © Maren Winter: 137; © Ekramar: 141
iStock: © dmilovanovic: 63; © DonNichols: 67; © AntiMartina: 69, back cover; © spline_x: 75; © karimitsu: 85; © emer1940: 105; © AlexRaths: 119
iStock/Getty Images: © dabjola: 93; © kaza-kovmaksim: 107; © Difydave: 115; © jopelka: 133; © sanatgen 135

10 9 8 7 6 5 4 3 2 1 0

Contents

Introduction

Not long after I appeared earthside, my parents had me outside foraging and enjoying nature. I couldn't even walk yet, but they carried me through the woods as they harvested morels, their favorite wild food. Growing up in the Missouri Ozarks, I spent most of my time outdoors enjoying the bounty nature had to offer. This region happens to have a lush supply of native medicinal (and edible) plants, mysterious crevices and caves to explore, and crystal clear creeks hiding hordes of crawdads and minnows. I love this area of the country so much that I still live here, on an 80-acre farm where I have plenty of room to grow and to wildcraft the plants I adore.

Since nature is my classroom, I decided my calling was to be an instructor. Teaching has always been a passion for me. In fact, I spent 10 years of my life teaching English in the Missouri public school system before retiring to teach the subjects I truly love: herbalism and aromatherapy. I became an American Herbalists Guild registered herbalist and founded my own online herb school, The Bitter Herb Academy. I spend most days talking with students and educating others on native medicinal plants. I also work to protect and preserve some of our threatened and endangered plants by showing how to grow these instead of harvesting them in the wild.

Through the years, I have used medicinal plants to help with a variety of conditions, ranging from skin rashes and wounds to anxiety and stress. I never cease to be amazed at how well they work to nourish and heal the body from the inside out. One of my most poignant memories is from 15 years ago, when I was diagnosed with a condition that causes my body to produce too much of a certain hormone. After some research, I decided to start taking vitex (chaste tree berry) tincture to see if this would help. Today, I have no more symptoms of this condition, and I'm healthier than ever. It's experiences like these that foster a strong reverence and passion in me when it comes to the capability of medicinal plants to heal the body. Not only have I experienced the healing potential of plants firsthand, I have watched over and over through the years as clients come to me raving about a plant I suggested for their condition. These remedies work, and with far fewer side effects than most pharmaceutical treatments.

If you're curious about this subject, it is my honor to empower and uplift you with this guide to medicinal plants. If you feel called to work with plants as I did many years ago, my hope is that this book will help guide and inspire you. Most of all, I want you to learn to approach this craft with confidence so you can reclaim the ancient knowledge our ancestors possessed about using plants to heal.

How to Use This Book

The format of *The Beginner's Guide to Medicinal Plants* is structured to help you get started in herbalism. Part 1 of this book will provide you with the basics, the foundational information you need to know, such as the history of herbal medicine, the gear and materials you'll need, how to harvest and process plants, and how to create beneficial formulations with the botanical treasures you've collected. Then in part 2, we'll put your know-how to use. I'll share detailed profiles of the 50 most essential medicinal plants, with instructions for creating my favorite teas, oils, tinctures, and other remedies and treatments. Soon you'll have a plant-based medicine cabinet that can handle everything from aches and pains to anxiety and stress.

Use part 2 not only to soothe and heal, but also to help you determine what plants you wish to work with. Read through all

50 profiles and see which ones appeal to your needs and aspirations. When you find a plant or remedy that calls to you, read about how to identify and harvest it in the wild as well as how to grow it at home. Perhaps most important, each profile instructs you on how to use the plant to create a powerful formulation. Read the instructions carefully and refer back to the preparation details in part 1 if you need to. Keep in mind that some treatments need extended time to infuse before they can be used, so you'll want to prepare them in advance. Don't forget to use the index in the back of the book to quickly browse the different plants discussed and find what you are looking for. Keep this book close, and feel free to stick it in your foraging backpack as you go exploring so you have a field guide handy!

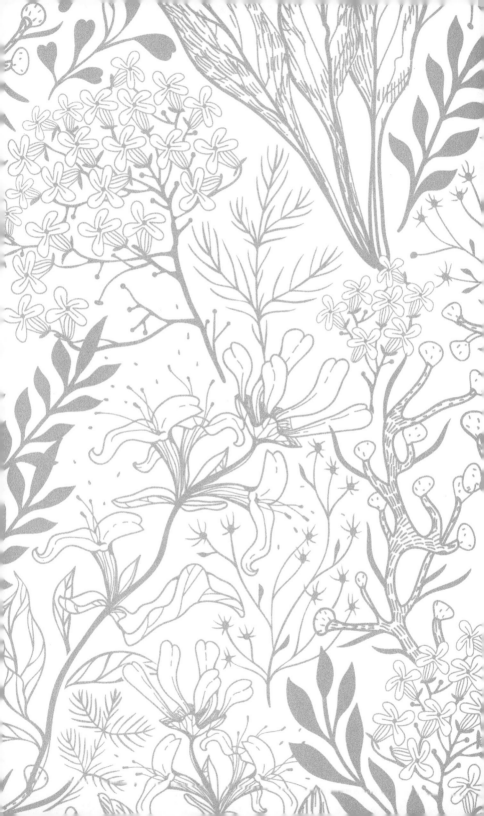

PART I

Plant Medicine 101

BEFORE GETTING TO KNOW THE PLANTS YOU WISH TO work with, you need to understand the basics of plant medicine itself. Working with medicinal plants enables you to discover and use their healing properties, as well as learn about the craft's rich history and beautiful traditions. In this first part of the book, we'll cover that and much more. You'll learn everything you need to know to get started using medicinal plants, including how to forage safely, how to harvest and prepare the plants you collect, and how to process them into various formulations, like salves and oil infusions.

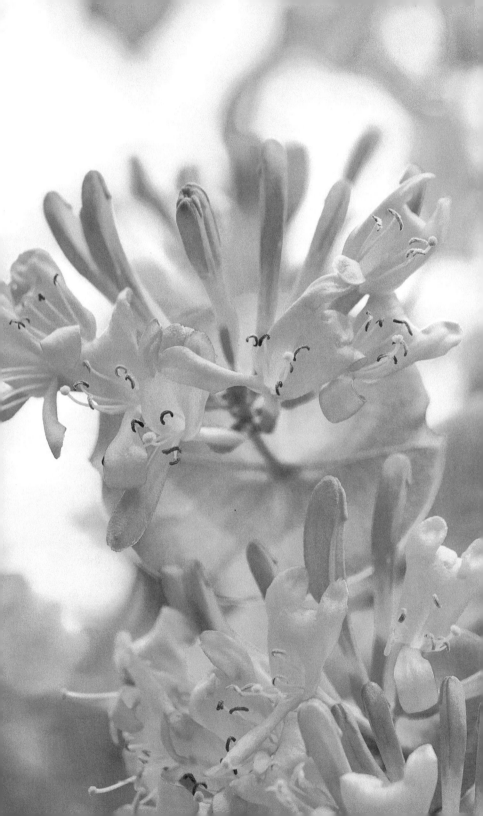

The Basics of Plant Healing

WELCOME TO THE VIBRANT AND EXCITING WORLD of plant medicine! In this chapter, we're going to start your voyage of discovery with the very basics by exploring what medicinal plants are, how they work in the body, and some of their many benefits. We'll also touch on the history and tradition of herbal medicine. The history of this craft is multifaceted and prolific, and learning more about it will help you understand the role of plant medicine more deeply. Along with that, we'll discuss how to choose the right plants and review what you need to get started harvesting them in the wild. All of this will help take the guesswork out of your herbal journey!

What Are Medicinal Plants?

As the name implies, a medicinal plant is one that contains therapeutic and healing chemical compounds that can have a positive effect on the human body. One could say that many medicinal plants work like pharmaceutical drugs; in fact, plants and pharmaceuticals are more closely related than many realize. Today, the pharmaceutical industry still uses plants to create a variety of common prescription and over-the-counter drugs. For instance, a popular pharmaceutical drug prescribed for influenza gets its main therapeutic compound, a chemical called "shikimic acid," from the spice star anise. That compound is also found in pine needles and unripe sweet gum tree seedpods. As another example, for centuries people have used white willow bark to treat various types of pain and fever. The active compound responsible for these medicinal effects is called "salicin." In modern times, this compound is broken down into salicylic acid to become the active ingredient in aspirin. There are countless examples of how plants are used to create pharmaceuticals many of us are familiar with.

The chemical compounds found in plants are called "phytochemicals." All plants contain a variety of these unique chemicals; medicinal plants often have one or two main phytochemicals that are responsible for their therapeutic effects. These phytochemical compounds, like the aforementioned salicin and shikimic acid, each act in different and specific ways in the human body to help foster healing.

The Benefits of Medicinal Plants

One of the things I appreciate most about medicinal plants is their ability to treat a condition gently yet effectively. I personally have never experienced nasty side effects when using a plant remedy. Nor have I experienced the "bandage effect," which means a drug or treatment merely acts as a bandage to cover up the symptoms instead of treating the root cause. I think many of us are so accustomed to using bandages to treat problems that we forget to dig deeper to figure out what is causing the issue in the first place. The trouble is, when one constantly masks symptoms, the condition could get much worse and even lead to other, more serious problems.

When using plant medicine, I have noticed that healing happens in a more holistic way. To be more precise, the *root cause is almost always addressed* and the problem goes away. Many holistic-minded people use medicinal plants for this reason. They wish to treat the body as a whole while addressing the root cause of the issue to achieve healing in the gentlest and most effective way possible.

A Supplement, Not a Replacement

There are times when it is acceptable to use an herbal remedy to treat a condition, and there are times when mainstream medicine is the appropriate avenue to treat illnesses, traumas, and other health issues. It is important to know when to use a plant remedy and when to seek medical help. Life doesn't have to be all or nothing; we don't have to choose one or the other. It is entirely possible to use both plant remedies and mainstream medicine to manage your health. There's no need to forgo medical treatment that may be very beneficial and lifesaving. Use good judgment when choosing when to see a doctor and when to use an herbal remedy. For example, some conditions can get much worse if they aren't treated aggressively and quickly. Certain infections need to be treated with antibiotics or they could spread and become life-threatening.

Never replace a prescription medication with a plant remedy, and always talk to your doctor before taking anything in order to avoid potential drug interactions. Some herbs and foods can interact with pharmaceutical medicines, so it is important to understand the risks and benefits of any herbal formulation before beginning a regimen. Many doctors are not trained in herbal medicine or the effects of plant remedies, so it may also be helpful to visit an integrative medicine physician who has training in both fields, in addition to speaking with your doctor.

The Long Tradition of Plant Medicine

Plant medicine spans time and is practiced around the globe. The use of plants to treat various conditions has been documented since humans were first able to record their experiences. The oldest written evidence of medicinal plants being used therapeutically has been found on a Sumerian clay slab from Nagpur and is about 5,000 years old. Before that, there's evidence that prehistoric humans were using plants medicinally as well.

Around the world, people of different regions use different approaches and methods to practice plant medicine. China has one of the world's oldest recorded plant medicine systems; Traditional Chinese Medicine (TCM) is at least 23 centuries old. This ancient system of medicine is still used today in China. In India, Ayurvedic medicine is still practiced. This system of medicine began around 1500 BC and has been written about in ancient books like the Atharvaveda, one of four ancient books of knowledge. The healing traditions of many Indigenous peoples include other rich and powerful systems of medicine that have been used for thousands of years. Since the dawn of civilization, many of these ancient practices, all of which include medicinal plant use, have served humankind well. And they continue to thrive as knowledge is passed from generation to generation.

How to Choose Plants for Medicine

Most herbalists will choose plants for clients (or themselves) based not only on the symptoms being presented, but also on other, more comprehensive principles. The important thing to keep in mind is that every person is different. What may work for one person may not work for another. This is because each person has a unique constitution and may react differently to the same plant remedy. Herbalists often look at more than just the symptoms. They take into consideration such things as diet, patterns of symptoms, and a patient's mental, physical, and emotional history. Treating the patient as a whole person instead of treating just a symptom or a disease is the cornerstone of being a good herbalist and using a good herbal protocol.

To better navigate these subtleties, herbal medicine practitioners often rely on the concept of energetics as well as the practice of choosing plants based on specific needs and physiological conditions. Though the details of them are beyond the scope of this book, let's look at how these ideas are implemented. As you deepen your involvement in plant medicine, I urge you to explore these concepts further.

Matching Energetics

Herbal energetics is one of several methods that can be used to match a remedy to a person. This concept is widely used in TCM. "Energetics" refers to the properties and actions of plants in the body. Each person can have a variety of different energetics as well: hot, cold, moist, or dry. Once these are determined, plants with matching energetics can be selected to complement the person's individual needs. Other factors that come into play include specific areas affected in the body, different therapeutic actions of each plant, addressing the root cause versus masking symptoms, and the availability of the plant being considered.

Plants for Specific Needs

As scientific research on different medicinal plants continues, we are learning more and more about how and why plants work in the body. For example, we know that compounds in echinacea affect the immune system in a specific way and have been shown to shorten the duration and lessen the symptoms of viral illness. And elderberry contains flavonoids that may suppress histamine production to help reduce inflammation. Being able to determine what plants will meet your need to treat a specific illness or injury depends on knowing about a wide variety of medicinal plants and their properties. This will take time, but the plants profiled in part 2 of this book are a perfect starting point for beginners.

What You Need to Get Started

In addition to the plants themselves, other materials will make your journey easier. Here's a list of helpful items to have on hand when growing, foraging, and processing medicinal plants.

A good spade. If you like growing herbs, you will need a spade for planting or transplanting. A spade is my best friend when it comes to digging up roots in the fall as well. The roots of several medicinal plants (like burdock, dandelion, and valerian) are the source of the plant's medicinal properties and should be harvested in the fall when the aerial (aboveground) parts have died away.

Areas for growing plants. I strongly feel that to fully understand and appreciate the plants you work with, you need to see and touch them as they grow and develop. Many medicinal plants can be grown in pots, so you don't need a lot of space. Since each plant has its own requirements, you'll need to match the space with the needs of the plants.

Scissors. These are very handy for harvesting a plant's aerial parts, especially leaves and flowers. They enable a clean break that doesn't harm the rest of the plant. You can purchase gardening scissors or herb scissors made for cutting plants, but I tend to use whatever I can find. Just keep your scissors sharp so you get a nice clean cut.

Drying materials. I use drying racks; these essentially are wooden frames with wire grids that you place the plants on to dry out and get airflow. You can also hang your plants in small bundles (from the ceiling, or somewhere out of the way) to dry them, or lay them on towels to dry. Some people use a food dehydrator, the kind that makes jerky and dehydrated vegetables. We'll talk more about the drying process in chapter 2.

Mortar and pestle. This kitchen and pharmacy tool set helps break down plants into powder. Another excellent option for this purpose is a good blender; I use my Vitamix.

Tins. Aluminum storage tins with lids work well for holding salves and tea blends.

Bottles and jars. I love using tinted dropper bottles in 1- and 2-ounce sizes to store tinctures and glycerites (fluid extracts made with glycerin). It's important to have larger heat-safe glass jars with lids on hand for storing dried herbs and making tinctures. I tend to hoard glass jars with lids for this purpose; our cabinets are full of repurposed sauce and jam jars!

Tea infusion tools. For making medicinal teas, you can buy empty tea bags to fill with tea blends of your choice; you can also use stainless steel infusers, which are perforated containers that can be filled with plants and placed in a cup of hot water.

Carrier oils. In chapter 3, you'll learn how carrier oils like olive and jojoba are used for making plant-infused oils.

Beeswax. Beeswax pellets are super handy for making salves. They melt fast and can be measured more precisely in liquid form.

Ethyl alcohol. Also known as ethanol, this is the kind of alcohol you can drink. I prefer at least 80 proof alcohol when making plant extracts called "tinctures," which you'll learn how to do in chapter 3. Vodka is an easily acquired and widely used option. If you don't wish to use alcohol, you can substitute apple cider vinegar or food-grade, non-GMO vegetable glycerin.

Double boiler. Another kitchen tool that's a real workhorse for preparing medical remedies, this is a must for making salves. It allows you to heat the ingredients gently, without damaging the delicate medicinal properties in beeswax.

When preparing to delve into herbalism, keep in mind that this is different from allopathic, or mainstream, medicine. There is no need to be fearful or apprehensive! You can do this, just as your ancestors have over the centuries.

KEY TAKEAWAYS

Now that you understand more about the history of plant medicine, you'll be ready to get your hands dirty in chapter 2! But first, here are some key points to keep in mind.

* Plants and pharmaceuticals are more closely related than many realize, and many pharmaceutical companies still use plants to make drugs today.

* Plants can gently yet effectively treat a condition thanks to compounds in each plant called "phytochemicals." Most medicinal plants have one or two active phytochemicals that are responsible for their effects.

* Medicinal plants have been used since before recorded history. Around the world, plant medicine has thrived for centuries with unique traditions and modalities in different cultures.

* Some items from the "What You Need to Get Started" list will prepare you to begin your plant medicine journey.

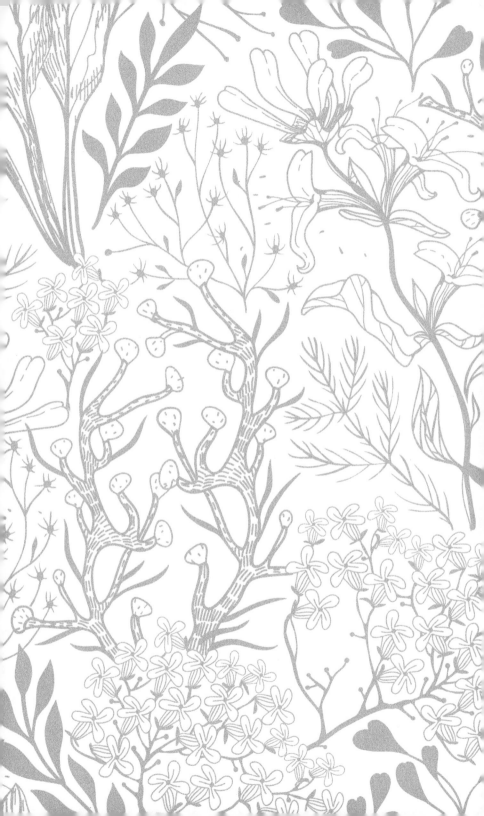

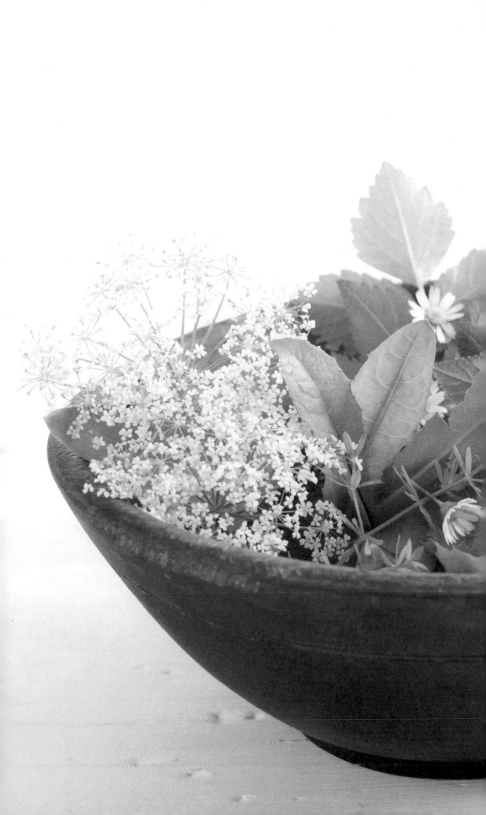

How to Grow and Forage for Medicinal Plants

OBTAINING QUALITY MEDICINAL HERBS IS THE cornerstone of creating effective herbal formulations. Over the years, I have found serious differences in potency, effectiveness, and overall strength depending on where I obtained the plants, when they were harvested, how they were processed, and even how they were stored. In this chapter, I will walk you through everything you need to know for growing, foraging, and purchasing the medicinal plants you wish to use to create remedies. And because the way that you store your plants matters, we'll also cover the dos and don'ts of proper herb processing and storage. To get the most out of your precious remedies, you need to know how to effectively store the plants themselves as well as the remedies you create. Soak up the knowledge in this chapter to reap the benefits of a successful medicine-making practice!

Growing Healing Herbs

Next to foraging, growing the plants I work with is my favorite way to ensure I have pure, quality organic materials to work with when creating remedies. When you grow your own plants, you get to see them in various stages of growth, which helps you learn more about them in an intimate way. Any method that allows you to physically handle, care for, and interact with the plants you use is the best way for you to learn and grow as an herbalist. If you feel you don't have a green thumb, don't let the idea of growing your own plants intimidate you! I have found that a great many of the plants I discuss in this book can easily be grown in pots, in raised beds, or even via sowing seeds in early spring. Most of these plants require little maintenance; they're not tropical houseplants that need constant care.

I have started plants from seed as well as purchased plants to transplant into my garden. Both methods have their pros and cons. Starting plants from seed can be super easy. I have an entire field of *Echinacea purpurea* as a result of throwing seeds whimsically into the air after my husband plowed up an area one spring. Certain plants just seem to take off easier and require little maintenance to get going. Some great plants that grow easily from seed include any plant in the mint family, echinacea (be patient, as it can take around two years for flowers to emerge), and calendula. Some plants do better if you purchase a small plant to transplant into a pot or raised bed. In my experience, these include passionflower (because the seeds need soaking before planting) and elderberry (it is easier to grow these from starters so you can get a bigger plant faster). Research each plant you wish to grow so you know which will do better in containers (calendula and lavender are great for growing in containers, as are all mints and herbs) or in the dirt outside. In addition to researching growing conditions, make sure you know which plants are unsafe for animals. For example, some mints, hops, eucalyptus, garlic, borage, and oregano can be toxic to pets if they are ingested in large amounts.

The Basics of Foraging

As previously stated, my favorite way to obtain medicinal plants is via foraging. After all, I am convinced that Mother Nature can do a better job growing a plant than I could any day. Plants foraged in the wild are often pure, haven't been sprayed with chemicals, and are available in abundance. Many of the plants I discuss later in this book can easily be found throughout North America, and many are very common as well as slightly invasive. This means you can harvest most of them without feeling guilty that you are damaging the ecosystem. This doesn't mean you shouldn't practice ethical foraging, though. Here are the principles to follow when you're out foraging.

Take only what you need. It is important to harvest only what you need for a remedy and leave the rest.

Take only 10 percent. If you happen to come across a stand of medicinal plants in the wild, a good rule of thumb is to take no more than 10 percent of what you found. In other words, leave 90 percent of what you see alone.

Consider the location. Never harvest plants from roadsides, as they can be polluted more than those in other locations, thanks to vehicle exhaust and roadside chemical spraying. Get permission and check local laws when foraging. Finally, never forage around power lines or railways, because these areas are sometimes sprayed heavily with chemicals.

Be safe. When foraging, keep safety in mind first and foremost. Always be aware of your surroundings and know what the risks of the local environment are, from ticks to bears to poison ivy. Keep abreast of weather conditions and bring whatever gear is necessary—map and compass, first aid kit, food, and water—anything that makes sense for the excursion you're taking.

Know what you're harvesting. Don't harvest any plant unless you are 100 percent sure you know what it is. Instead, take pictures of unknown plants with your phone so you can research and get a positive ID. I like some plant identification apps, but I sometimes find them to be way off, so I always cross-reference the results with other sources, books, and field guides to make sure. You can use this book to help identify plants in the field, as it contains clear photos and descriptions of many medicinal plants you will likely come across. Be patient! Put in the work and eventually certain plants will seem like familiar old friends.

Identifying Edible and Medicinal Plants

You can identify plants by taking a closer look at their stems, leaves, flowers, and fruit, as well as any other interesting characteristics you notice. Take clear pictures of each, because you never know what might be helpful. For example, did you know that most mint species have square stems? If you find a plant in the wild with a square stem, chances are it is in the mint family, which may help you narrow things down a bit.

Flowers can be a great identifying feature because they stand out with their unique colors and shapes. Count the petals and take note of the overall flower shape to narrow down identification options.

Leaves can be key for IDing a plant because they come in a variety of hues, can have smooth or toothed edges, and come in a variety of shapes.

Fruit can be a dead giveaway as well. For example, it can be hard to find red raspberry leaves to harvest for tea, but it is easier to spot the plant once the berries appear.

Don't forget that smell can play a big role in identification, especially when identifying famously aromatic herbs like mints and valerian root. Take notes or use your phone to record a description of a plant's aroma.

The Universal Edibility Test

Suppose you're out in the field foraging and you want to know if a plant is edible or not. Obviously, just taking a bite out of it is *not* the right move. Always keep in mind the universal foraging rule: *Don't eat anything you cannot identify 100 percent.* Second, avoid eating plants with certain characteristics: milky sap; white or yellow berries; thorns; umbrella-shaped flower heads (also called "umbels"); shiny leaves; beans, bulbs, or seeds that grow in pods; leaves in groups of three (poison ivy); a bitter or soapy flavor; or anything that appears rotten or "off." Also avoid plants with a bitter or almondlike smell.

One interesting method for assessing edibility, described in *The U.S. Army Survival Manual,* is the Universal Edibility Test. This calls for you to first fast for eight hours before testing a plant, and to continue fasting during the test. With that in mind, here's how it works:

The first step is to separate the plant into five parts: roots, stem, leaves, buds, and flowers. Some plants have edible and nonedible parts, so each of these parts should be tested separately.

Perform a contact test by crushing up one part of the plant and rubbing it on the inside of your elbow or wrist for 10 to 15 minutes. Check for signs of a skin reaction, such as redness, hives, welts, bumps, or stinging. Consider any reaction to be a sign that the tested part is inedible.

The next step is to cook each part of the plant. There are many plants that aren't good for you to eat raw but can be eaten if cooked. Take each part (after cooking) and press it to your lips for 3 minutes. Watch for signs of a reaction. If you don't have a reaction, that part may be edible.

The last step is to taste the plant by placing a small piece in your mouth. Hold it on your tongue for 15 minutes before chewing. If you don't notice a reaction (such as tingling, burning, etc.) you can chew the plant, and then hold it in your mouth for another 15 minutes to watch for reactions. Spit the plant out immediately if you notice any burning, numbness, tingling, or other signs of a reaction. Rinse your mouth with water as well.

If a portion of a plant passes all these tests, it may be safe to swallow. It is advisable not to eat anything else for another 8 hours following swallowing, to ensure that any effects are due to the plant. If you feel sick to your stomach or start vomiting, drink plenty of water. If you don't notice any adverse symptoms, the plant is likely edible, and you can eat more.

You may not be in a position to use this elaborate test anytime soon. But it certainly demonstrates the need for caution with ingesting plants you don't know anything about. Remember, the Universal Edibility Test should be used as Plan B: Even safe plants in this book may not pass all the criteria for the test. Plan A should be an affirmative identification.

Buying Medicinal Plants

You may want to work with plants that you can't find in the wild, in which case buying the dried herbs is an option. Personally, I'm very picky about purchasing herbs. Here are some considerations to help you find the best-quality products.

Know how they were harvested. If the plants you're purchasing have been wildcrafted (harvested from the wild), look for a company that practices ethical and sustainable harvesting. It's important to know the date the plant was collected as well, because time deteriorates potency. I choose plants that have been harvested and dried as recently as possible and avoid plants that are over 1 year old.

Inspect the product. If possible, check the color; if the plants appear pale and bleached, avoid purchasing them. In addition to this, I have learned to double-check which parts of the plant I am purchasing. For example, I bought calendula from a reputable company once, and when I opened the bag, I was shocked to see pale yellow petals and no intact flowers. When purchasing calendula, I want to see the whole flower, with the resinous and medicinal bract attached.

Know how they were prepared. The vendor should specify how the plants were dried. I personally do not purchase plants that have been dried with a dehydrator. That can expose the plants to too much heat too quickly, which decreases the potency and deteriorates certain phytochemicals that make plants beneficial.

Look for organic. I prefer certified organically grown herbs so I know they haven't been sprayed with pesticides or other chemicals.

Preserving and Storing Your Medicinal Plants

Once I harvest my medicinal plants, I wish to keep them as potent and fresh as possible. How we preserve and store our herbs makes a big difference! Another important task is labeling our plant material to make sure we know what we have and can find what we need. In these next pages, you'll learn how to properly dry, store, and label the various plants and plant remedies you work with. These key practices will ensure you have the best products possible!

Drying

Most of the herbs I harvest will be dried; drying preserves the plants so we can use them to make medicine when we choose, instead of having to do it as soon as we collect them. Not all herbs should be dried; some plants, like chickweed, St. John's wort, and cleavers, are best prepared when they are fresh for a better product. (The profiles in part 2 will tell you which preparations require fresh or dried plants.) But most remedies call for dried plant material. Here are some options.

Use a rack. Drying racks are my favorite way to dry the plants; it's a simple method that allows them to dry gently, without the use of added heat that can damage certain phytochemicals. I place my racks in a room of my house that has good airflow and ventilation, and the plants are nicely dried within a few days. Herb and plant drying racks are inexpensive and easily obtained; you can even make your own by adding a screen or mesh to a wooden frame.

Hang 'em up. Another option is to hang the plants in small bundles from the ceiling. Don't make the bundles too thick, or they won't get good airflow and may develop mold. And don't dry plants in direct sunlight; the UV rays from the sun will damage important compounds in the plants needed for maximum medicinal effect.

Use a towel. For small batches, you can spread a towel on a counter or tabletop. Simply lay the plants on the towel and give them a few days to dry out.

Plants are fully dried when they have a lightly crispy texture and are not soft anymore. They should still retain their vibrant color and not appear pale or bleached. When they are fully dried, I place the plants in glass jars for storage and keep these jars in a dark cabinet, where no sunlight can damage the plants.

Labeling

Even the most experienced herbalists sometimes forget to properly label their dried plants or herbal formulations. This is a bad habit, because you may not be able to identify or remember the contents of a container after some time has passed. Trust me, having to throw out perfectly good plants or remedies due to improper labeling is downright painful! Save yourself the pain.

For plants I have dried, I label the jar or container with the name of the plant and when it was harvested. As a rule, I try to use all my dried plants within one year. It is entirely possible to use your dried herbs after a year has passed, but I cannot guarantee their potency.

For remedies, I write the name of the plant on the label, along with the type of formulation (tincture, tea, tonic, etc.), the date the plant was harvested, the expiration date of the formulation (if applicable), and the dosage.

You can purchase labels for your storage containers or simply write on a piece of tape with a Sharpie. Any method that produces a lasting, legible label is fine. Just don't forget to do it!

Preserving Herbal Preparations

Where to keep your remedies once you've prepared and labeled them? Here are some guidelines.

Tinctures. There is a reason that tinctures are one of my favorite ways to process medicinal plants. Tinctures—alcohol-based plant extracts—last a lot longer than many other herbal preparations, due to their alcohol content. Alcohol not only makes a great solvent to pull medicinal compounds from plants, but it also helps preserve the plants. I store my tinctures in tinted bottles to protect them from potentially damaging sunlight, and I keep them in a cool, dark area of my house. This usually consists of a large cabinet I have in my basement, with doors I can shut to keep out light. When stored properly, tinctures can last up to seven years, and maybe even longer.

Oils and salves. I keep these in a closed cabinet as well, as this is a cool, dark space with a stable temperature. It is important to make sure the area you choose to store your formulations has a stable temperature. Fluctuating temperatures can damage your product.

Water-based preparations. For infusions, teas, and other water-based remedies, I have a designated spot in my refrigerator. Water-based preparations with no fixatives will only last a few days to a week in the refrigerator. To further preserve these, you can pour them into ice cube trays and freeze them overnight. Pop them out and store them in a labeled freezer bag to thaw as needed.

KEY TAKEAWAYS

Whether you decide to grow, forage, or purchase your herbs, effective remedies require knowing how to store and preserve them so you can create something truly magnificent and valuable. Keep the following in mind as you deepen your knowledge of plant medicine.

❀ Growing your own plants is a great way to learn about them and build your stock of plant material for remedies. Some plants are easy to grow from seed; others are best grown from a small starter.

❀ Keep safety and sustainability in mind while foraging. Don't collect more than 10 percent of what you find.

❀ After harvesting your plants, dry them on racks, on a towel, or by hanging them from the ceiling in small bundles. Make sure the drying area has sufficient airflow.

❀ Preserving your plants and plant remedies properly is essential. Keep plants and remedies out of the sunlight and keep the temperature stable. Water-based remedies need to be refrigerated or frozen promptly. Label everything!

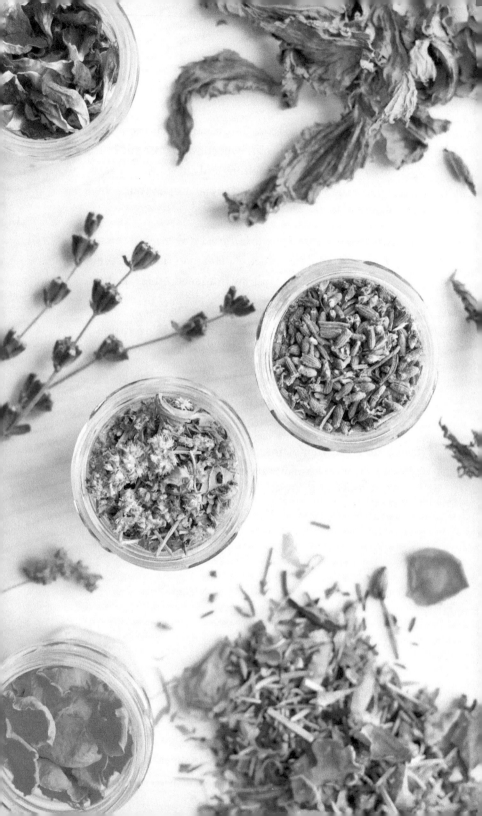

Basic Techniques for Using Medicinal Plants

THERE ARE A LOT OF WAYS TO USE MEDICINAL PLANTS.
All the possibilities can be kind of intimidating for
someone new to herbal medicine, but never fear! Now
that you know how to harvest and store your plants, it's
time to create the remedies you've been working toward.
This chapter will delve into the most common herbal
preparation methods so you can approach the craft
feeling confident and empowered. In addition to learning
how to make various herbal remedies, you will learn the
best way to use them so you can get the most out of the
precious remedies you create.

Common Preparations of Plant Medicine

I love the fact that there are different ways to prepare herbal medicine, because it reminds me that over the centuries humans have discovered that the way a medicinal plant is prepared matters. Some plants work better in water-soluble solutions, and other plants do better in alcohol-soluble ones. Some are best taken as teas; others work well if applied to the skin in a salve. Some plants need a little heat to help make a stronger remedy, whereas others will be rendered less effective with added heat. When researching each plant that you grow, wildcraft, or purchase, make sure you research which herbal preparation is best to get the most out of that particular plant. (For the plants profiled in the second part of this book, the research has been done for you.) Here are some common herbal preparations and how to create them.

A note about sterilization: Some preparations call for you to use a sterile jar or container. Many dishwashers have a "sterilize" setting that hits the contents with hot steam. That's one way to sterilize your preparation materials. If you don't have that available, you can boil some water in a pot and place the container in there for a few minutes, and then remove it with tongs. This prevents mold or another contaminant from taking hold in your remedies. Always discard any remedy that shows signs of mold, especially water-based remedies, even if they haven't reached their expiration date.

Teas

Teas are beverages made by infusing plant material in hot water. Teas can include blends of various roots, leaves, flowers, or bark from a medicinal or edible plant. In the UK, herbal teas are called "tisanes," a term you may encounter in your research. This popular method of administrating herbal medicine has been used since humankind discovered medicinal plants. Teas are easy and quick to make; I keep plenty of tea bags on hand, as well as those handy stainless steel tea infusion devices, so I can make tea as I need it.

The basic method is probably familiar to you if you're a tea drinker: Heat a cup of water (it doesn't have to be boiling) and then place the tea bag or infusion device, filled with plant material, into the water. Allow 10 to 15 minutes for the tea to infuse. Then remove the bag or infuser, add raw honey if you'd like, and wait for your cup of medicinal goodness to cool down enough to drink.

Tinctures

Tinctures are one of my favorite ways to prepare medicinal plants. I love them for two reasons: one, they are super easy to make; and two, they last for years! Tinctures are simply herbal extracts made by infusing plant material into ethyl alcohol (aka ethanol, the kind of alcohol you can drink). I prefer using at least 80 proof alcohol for tinctures. Many herbalists use vodka, which is inexpensive and easy to find. I also like that it's clear, which enables me to watch as the plants change the hue of the liquid over time. The higher proof alcohol also helps preserve the tincture and makes a strong herbal preparation. Most tinctures last up to seven years, but I have many in my apothecary that are much older, and they are still as strong as ever.

You can use fresh or dried plants to make a tincture. I'll share many of my favorite preparations in part 2, but the basic process is to fill a sterile glass jar with the plant material, cover it completely in alcohol, and allow this mixture to infuse for four to six weeks in a cool, dark place. Shake your tincture jar daily to further promote infusion. After the four to six weeks have passed, strain out the liquid and bottle it in labeled dropper bottles. You don't have to refrigerate these; just make sure they sit in a cool, temperature-stable place out of direct sunlight.

Tonics and Syrups

You may see an herbal remedy described as a "tonic," which sounds like a type of preparation. But tonic is actually a term describing an herb or blend of herbs that works to tone, restore, or rejuvenate the body. Tonics are included in many herbal preparations. Most are water-based, but some can have alcohol, vinegar, or other liquids added. There is no firm rule for how a tonic is prepared.

An herbal syrup is made by boiling the plant material in water until it creates a more concentrated liquid, then straining out solids and adding sugar or raw honey for a sweet, syrupy consistency. I personally don't use processed sugar in my syrups because I believe this is counterintuitive to healing. I use a small amount of raw honey sometimes, as raw honey has medicinal properties of its own. Syrups have a high water content and so should be refrigerated and used within three to six months.

Nourishing Herbal Infusions

Herbal infusions are essentially more strongly brewed herbal teas used for their medicinal benefits. These are great for people who need something stronger than a tea for their predicament. As a general rule, infusions are made by boiling a quart of water on the stove. While the water is coming to a boil, fill a quart mason jar with one ounce of dried and chopped plant material (use one ounce for every quart of water used). When the water has come to a boil, carefully pour it into the quart jar over the plant matter. Since the water is boiling, it's important to use a mason jar or another jar that can withstand the heat.

Place a lid on the jar and allow this to infuse for several hours. I like to make mine before bed and then let the material infuse throughout the night. The next morning, I strain out the mix, bottle the liquid, and refrigerate it. For most infusions, you should drink one to three cups each day, depending on what herbs you use. Because this is a water-based remedy, it doesn't have a long shelf life and should be used within three to five days.

Oils

Herb-infused oils are great for nourishing the skin and healing various skin conditions. They're usually applied directly to the affected area. There are two main ways to make an herb-infused oil.

The first is to fill a sterile mason jar with dried plant material (only use dried herbs to make an oil infusion, as any water content can result in mold over time), then completely cover the plant material with a carrier oil. Some great carrier oils include jojoba oil, olive oil, sweet almond oil, grapeseed oil, and hempseed oil. Place a lid on the jar and sit it in a cool, dark place for four to six weeks, shaking the jar daily to promote infusion. Then strain the oil through a cheesecloth and bottle your herb-infused oil.

The other method is to fill the jar with plant material, cover it in a carrier oil, and then sit this in a pan of warm to hot water (use the burner's "warm" or lowest setting). Make sure the water level in the pan is high enough to cover most of the oil in the jar, but not so high that it will spill into the jar. Let this infuse with the lid off for up to eight hours. Sometimes I allow the mixture to infuse much longer, depending on the plant I am working with and how strong I want the infusion to be. Then strain the oil and bottle it.

Store herb-infused oils in a cool, temperature-stable place, out of direct sunlight. Check the expiration date on the bottle of carrier oil you use, as this will be the expiration date you need to follow for your herb-infused oil. Massage or apply herb-infused oils into the skin as needed for healing.

Poultices and Compresses

Herbal poultices are a quick and handy way to use a plant for healing the skin. To make one, simply mash up a fresh herb and apply it directly to a bug bite, sting, wound, or injury. If using a dried herb, you can add a tiny amount of water and mix with a mortar and pestle until you reach a consistency you like. Reapply these as often as needed.

Herbal compresses take a little longer to prepare. To make one, boil a few teaspoons or tablespoons (it depends on the plant you are working with) of the plant material in a few cups of water for fifteen to twenty minutes. Once the water has cooled a bit, dip a clean cloth into the solution (dish towels and old clothes cut into rags are good for this). Wring out the cloth a bit and apply it to wounds, rashes, or painful areas to promote relief. These can be administered warm or cold, depending on the situation; for a cold compress, refrigerate the liquid for a while before use. You can keep soaking up liquid and reapplying it to the area as often as you want, or until the liquid is gone. Try to use up the liquid within two to three days, and refrigerate it between uses.

Dosage and Administration

Safe dosage matters, so it is important to start off small and work your way up to a dose that suits you and your needs. Always start with the smallest recommended dosage of an herbal remedy, and if you don't feel relief after a while, you can go up to a larger dose. Some people find that they only need a small amount of a tincture or infusion to feel better and manage their condition, whereas others find that they need more to achieve a therapeutic effect. Dosage will vary depending on the plant used, as well as the type of herbal preparation you are using. For example, a tea is not as strong as a tincture; you wouldn't want to drink a cup of tincture like you do tea.

As a general rule, most tincture dosages range from a few drops to a few dropperfuls. (A "dropperful" of a tincture is around 30 drops.)

Most teas call for 1 to 3 or more cups daily depending on the herb used and the issue being treated.

Infusion doses can range from 1 to 3 or more cups daily as well.

Syrups are usually taken in small or moderate doses (like 1 teaspoon to 1 tablespoon) because they are very sweet and sugary.

Topical applications like salves, oil, poultices, and compresses are often used as needed, and in whatever amount you feel is necessary for the issue.

Salves

Herbal salves are simply oil infusions that have beeswax added to achieve a thicker consistency. Salves tend to be easier to apply to the skin and less messy. They stay in place better than oil to help heal wounds, rashes, and the like faster. As a general rule, a salve can be made by blending 1 ounce of beeswax pellets with 8 ounces of herb-infused oil. Start by melting the beeswax in the top of a double boiler—fill the bottom halfway to three-quarters with water, and bring to a boil. Add herb-infused oil to the beeswax once it has fully melted. Blend this together well, add 5 to 10 drops of essential oils if you want, and then pour into jars or tins to cool. Store your salves in a cool area, because they can melt easily if they are left in a warm spot for too long. Apply a salve as often as you want to nourish, heal, or protect the skin.

The Power of Herbs

Over the years, I have come to appreciate and adore what medicinal plants have done for me and my family. I have watched with amazement as they have healed my children, myself, and my community in times of need. It never gets old having someone come up to me and tell me how much of a difference a remedy has made in their life. It leaves me feeling empowered and grateful that I chose this line of work.

All those benefits and more await you as you begin your own explorations into herbal medicine. You'll find yourself connected to a tradition that began before recorded history and is supported by the latest scientific investigations. You'll see the world around you in a new way as you come to identify dozens, and then hundreds, of wild-growing plants that you never noticed before. And you'll feel the amazement that comes from witnessing how much healing power exists in the natural world, if we only hear the wisdom passed on to us by those who came before. Are you excited to see where this journey will take you? Let's find out!

KEY TAKEAWAYS

- There are many types of herbal preparations you can make, depending on your needs and the plants you wish to work with.

- Some common herbal preparations include teas, tinctures, infusions, syrups, oils, poultices, compresses, and salves.

- Dosage varies depending on the preparation you made, the issue you wish to address, and the plants you are working with.

- To be on the safe side, always start with the lowest recommended dosage, then work your way up if needed.

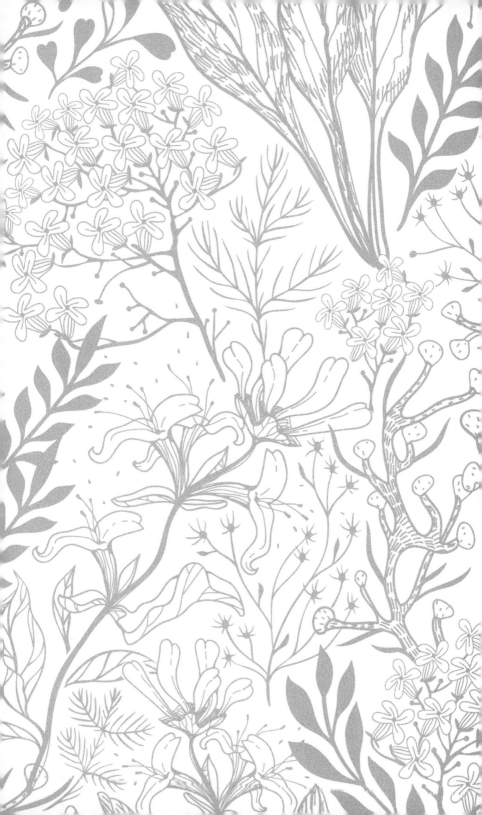

PART II

The 50 Most Essential Medicinal Plants

"WHERE DO I START?" IS A QUESTION I'M OFTEN ASKED by people who want to become involved in herbal medicine. Well, in these next pages, I'm giving you not one, but 50 possible starting points!

Now that you've gotten started, learning about the plants and how to identify them is the true first step. Gathering them, whether during a hike in the woods or from a garden bed in your backyard, sets everything in motion. Properly drying and storing (and don't forget labeling!) your plant material ensures you have the most potent components to work with. Part of the joy of herbal medicine is knowing that you've been the hands-on director of the whole process, from raw materials to final product.

That said, creating the remedies is the end goal, right? I'm excited to share with you my 50 favorite medicinal plants, along with the 50 most essential remedies that every herbalist will want in their inventory. I suggest you read through this whole list first, then begin with a few plants that catch your interest. Read the instructions carefully; if needed, refer back to chapter 3 (page 27) for more details about the preparations. Now on to the plants!

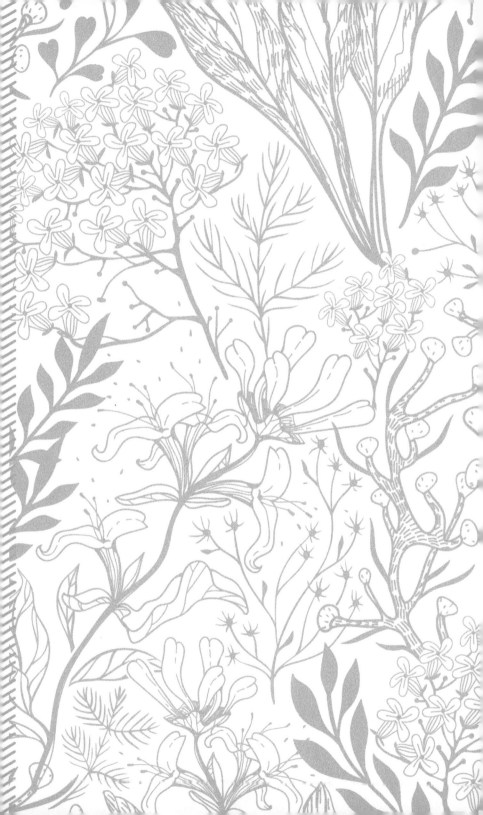

50
Essential
Medicinal
Plants

Agrimony

I first noticed this plant on my homestead because the little spikes covered in yellow flowers caught my attention; it likes to grow at the wood's edge in the summer months. As a mom, I've found agrimony to come in handy a time or two, because it helps with digestive issues like mild diarrhea, nausea, vomiting, and irritable bowel issues. The reason it works so well is because its compounds are astringent and anti-inflammatory, helping to calm spastic bowels while also coating the lining of the digestive tract to provide relief. Other historic uses of agrimony include chewing it to eliminate mouth sores and sore throats. Some Indigenous peoples used agrimony as a blood purifier (that is, to eliminate toxins) as well as to treat diarrhea and vomiting. Agrimony is a gentle remedy, safe enough for use by adults and children alike. I collect all its aerial parts to make tea. Simply harvest the plant, dry it, and store in an airtight glass jar to have on hand when you need it.

Find the Agrimony remedy on page 144.

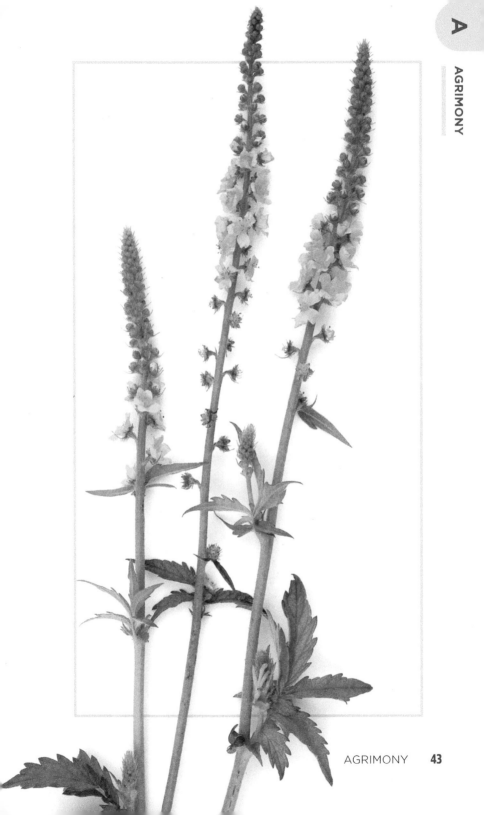

Boneset

This North American plant can be found in fields and meadows throughout the summer months and into autumn. Boneset wasn't named for a miraculous ability to set bones or anything of that nature. It got its unique name for its ability to bring down high fevers and relieve muscle and joint pain that resulted from a condition called "breakbone fever." This is a viral, mosquito-borne illness also known as "dengue fever." Boneset can work to bring down fevers by inducing sweating, a property that several plants possess (we herbalists refer to these as "febrifuge" plants). In addition, boneset is very useful for treating a wide range of minor viral infections. It can also help amplify the immune system's response to a virus or infection so the body can fight it off faster. Some Indigenous peoples used this plant for centuries to treat any illness that presented with a fever, long before its healing powers were well known across the world. I love to combine this plant with echinacea or elderberry when making medicinal preparations. The ingredients seem to work on many levels in synergy to tackle a virus or infection.

Find the Boneset remedy on page 145.

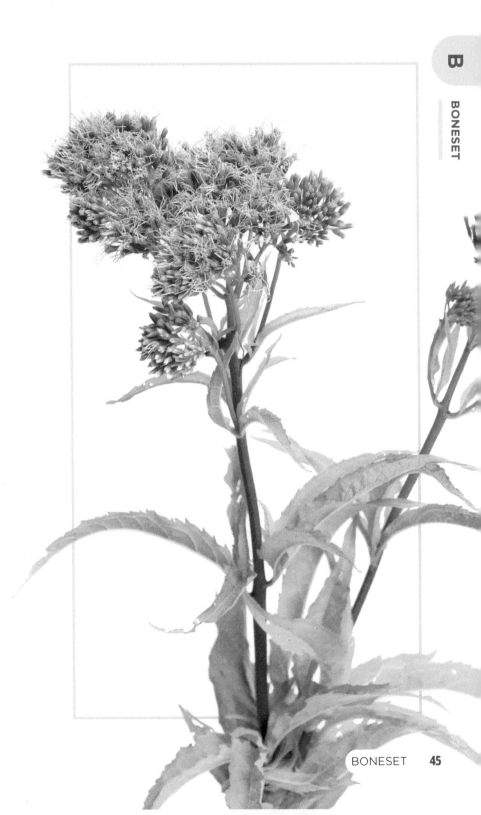

Burdock

Burdock can be found blooming from June to October in North America, though it's only in its second year of growth that it develops a stem and grows tall. The blooms are noticeable because the flowers have a thistlelike appearance and are a lovely shade of purple. You may know burdock as the plant that leaves sticky burrs all over your clothes when you walk beside it. The root of this plant has been used historically for medicinal purposes; it's packed with antioxidants that help eliminate potentially dangerous free radicals from the body. These also work to reduce inflammation in the body. The root—which should be harvested in the autumn of the first-year growth, or in the second year before the stem appears—has widely been used as a blood purifier. That is, it's known for its ability to remove toxins from the bloodstream. Not only has burdock root been shown to detoxify the blood, but it can also help improve circulation. Because it can help cleanse the body from impurities, burdock can be a very effective remedy for supporting the liver and healing the body from the inside out. The effects of taking burdock root on a regular basis can particularly be seen on the skin: Acne can disappear, as can skin conditions like eczema. In addition to internal use, burdock root has been used externally to treat wounds, burns, and other skin trauma.

Find the Burdock remedy on page 146.

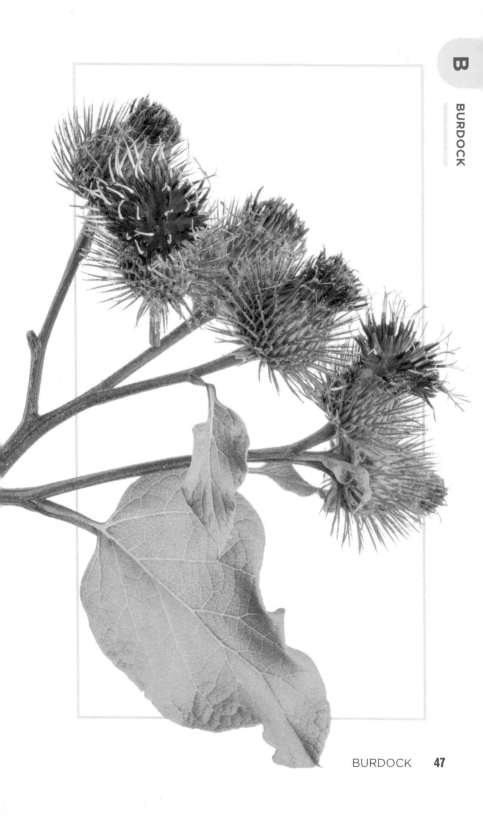

Calendula

I could stare at my calendula-infused oil all day! The vibrant orange-gold color of this flower infuses into a carrier oil to create a truly beautiful remedy that can heal a variety of skin conditions. Calendula is often called the "pot marigold" because it can easily be grown in containers. Despite the similar color, don't confuse this plant with common marigold, as it is a different plant altogether. If purchasing, check for the Latin name for this plant, *Calendula officinalis*. Calendula has been used historically for both internal and external health issues. It can be infused in hot water to make a tea for digestive health, lymphatic support, and inflammation reduction. Externally, it is handy for treating wounds, infections (both bacterial and fungal), inflammation, irritations, burns, and all kinds of rashes. Since I tend to be accident-prone, I like to have calendula oil on hand to massage into bumps, bruises, and other minor injuries. As a mom of two active little boys, I have used calendula since their birth to treat diaper rashes, eczema, fungal rashes, and more. It is a genuine staple in my natural medicine cabinet.

Find the Calendula remedy on page 147.

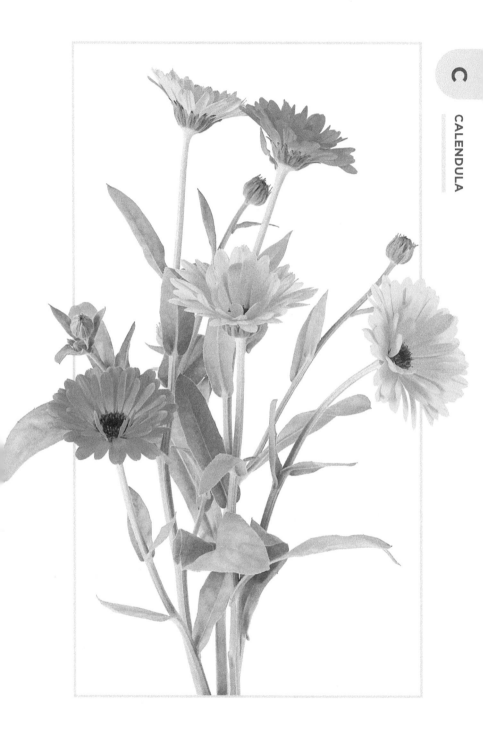

California Poppy

These flowers are a bright and lovely shade of orange-yellow. The frilly leaves are a unique shade of green-blue. In some areas of California, there are whole mountainsides and meadows full of California poppies. This poppy is actually the California state flower! Just because they are native to California doesn't mean they cannot grow anywhere else, though. These are a favorite of many gardeners for their beauty and effortless growing abilities. Note that though these gorgeous and sunny plants are technically poppies, they do not in any way have the same compounds that the opium poppy possesses. They do, however, have gentle nervine (nerve soothing) and sedative properties that can relieve nerve pain, calm headaches, and soothe anxiety and insomnia. California poppy has long been used in children as well to treat bed wetting, restlessness, overexcitement, and nervous agitation. The aerial parts are used medicinally.

Find the California Poppy remedy on page 148.

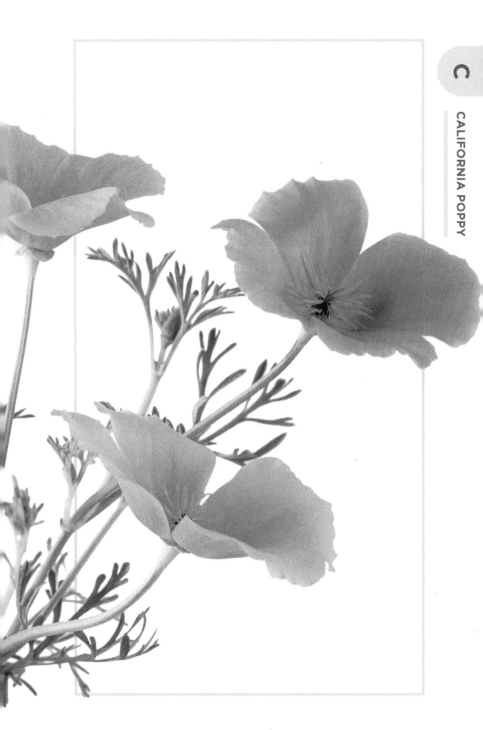

Catnip

This member of the mint family is a lighter shade of green than other mints; it tends to appear grayish-green. It has pale pink to white flowers on top and a pleasant, minty aroma. Just because catnip is famous for making our feline friends go wild doesn't mean it has the same effect on humans. In fact, it has the opposite effect! Instead of stimulating and exciting humans, catnip calms the mind and body. It is a gentle yet powerful herb for bringing peace and tranquility. And it's safe enough for children and adults alike. We can infuse 2 teaspoons of dried and chopped catnip in a cup of water to make a calming tea that is great for insomnia, restlessness, and overstimulation. Catnip has been used (mostly in tea form) to treat intestinal cramps, digestive issues, menstrual issues, diarrhea, colic, viruses, and fevers. If pregnant, avoid catnip in excessive amounts as it can stimulate the uterus to promote menstruation. It may also relieve aches, pains, and sore muscles when used as a compress. One of my favorite uses for catnip is to bring down high fevers and gently cool the body during sickness.

Find the Catnip remedy on page 149.

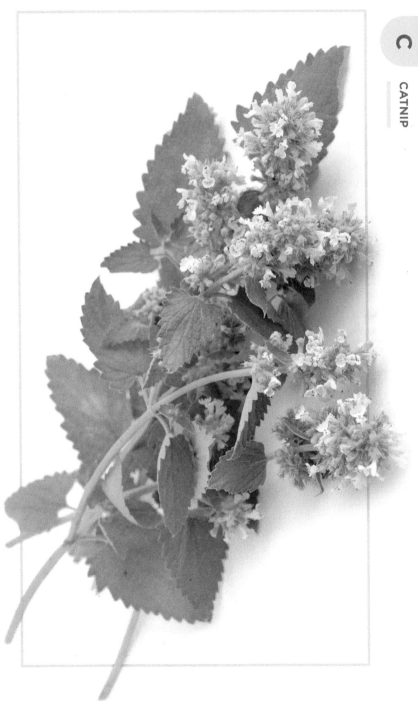

Cayenne

You may know cayenne as a pepper that adds a spicy kick to food dishes, but this little red pepper happens to contain medicinal properties. Its secret is a compound called "capsaicin," which can block pain in the nerves as well as relieve inflammation. Capsaicin is also an effective compound for stimulating blood circulation to support the heart and cardiovascular system. Remedies with cayenne have been used to treat blood circulation issues, cardiac arrhythmia, and heart palpitations. They have also been used externally on areas of the body that aren't getting the blood circulation they need. Cayenne is a friend to other herbal remedies because its circulation-stimulating effects allow remedies to function more efficiently in the body. I make a lovely red salve with cayenne that can be massaged into the legs, arms, or other areas of the body needing more circulation. I also find it very helpful for sore joints and painful areas.

Find the Cayenne remedy on page 150.

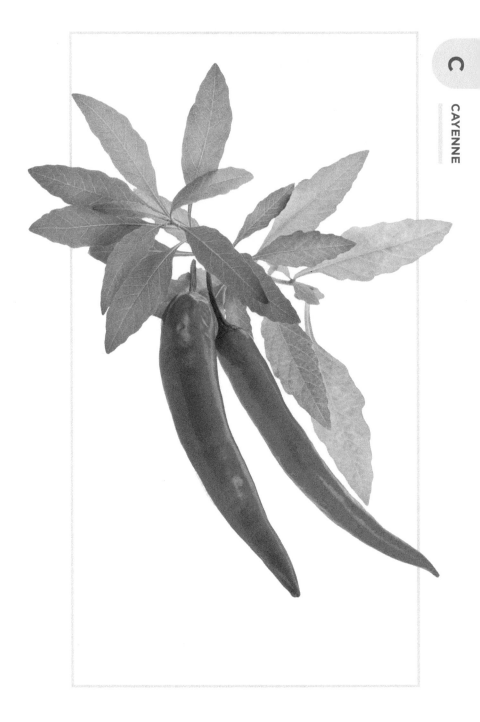

Chamomile

There are two main species of chamomile: German chamomile (*Matricaria chamomilla*) and Roman chamomile (*Chamaemelum nobile*). Both have similar characteristics, with Roman chamomile being especially known for its calming properties as well as its ability to help relieve aches, pains, and spasmodic conditions. The flowers and leaves of this species tend to be thicker and larger than German chamomile. Chamomile is known for its nervine (nerve calming) and sedative properties. It is also used to calm digestive upset. Just as both chamomile species can calm the nerves when taken internally, they can also calm externally by soothing irritated and inflamed skin. They may help improve skin tone by reducing redness, blotchiness, and irritation. And their antimicrobial properties help calm acne and gently restore pH balance for all skin types. Chamomile is one of my favorite plants for promoting beautiful, clear skin. Do not use chamomile if you have allergies to plants in the aster family, one of the biggest plant families in the world, which includes asters, sunflowers, daisies, marigolds, and zinnias. Chamomile's appearance is commonly confused with daisies and fleabane, so study carefully for correct identification.

Find the Chamomile remedy on page 151.

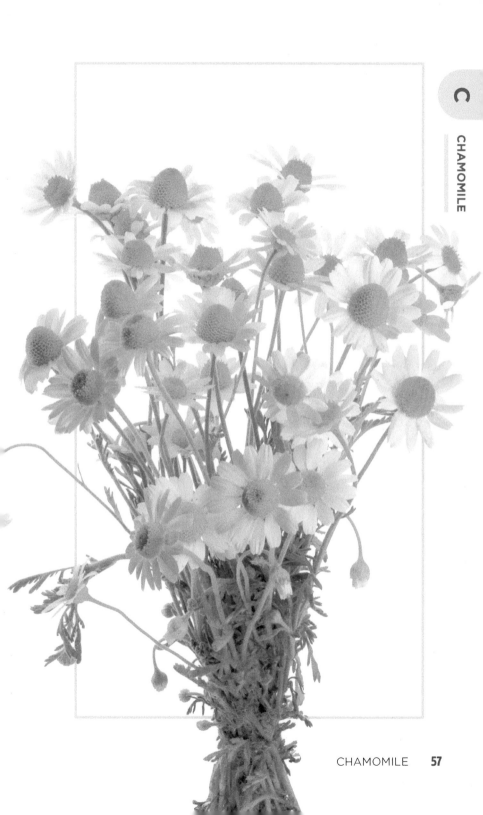

Chickweed

Look carefully in your yard during the spring and fall months, and you are likely to find this unassuming green plant. Chickweed is very common throughout most of North America. Its tiny white flowers look like little stars, and its diminutive leaves are shaped somewhat like hearts. Chickweed doesn't get very tall, and when it does, it tends to spread on the ground. Because this plant prefers cooler weather, it may die away in the summer and come back again in the fall. Don't be fooled by its size! This little botanical packs a big punch when it comes to healing red, irritated, and inflamed skin rashes. It makes the perfect remedy for conditions like eczema, diaper rash, and heat rash. Chickweed is known for its gentle, cooling effect that soothes angry skin. Harvest what you can in the spring so you have this remedy ready in the summer months, as heat tends to cause rashes and skin inflammation. Chickweed isn't just amazing for skin issues; it's also effective for treating gastrointestinal issues, because it can soothe and calm intestinal membranes. Simply infuse a teaspoon or two of the plant in a hot cup of water to make tea for irritable bowel syndrome (IBS) or gastrointestinal upset. Have a cup or two daily to tackle intestinal spasms and other issues that cause digestive problems.

Find the Chickweed remedy on pages 152–153.

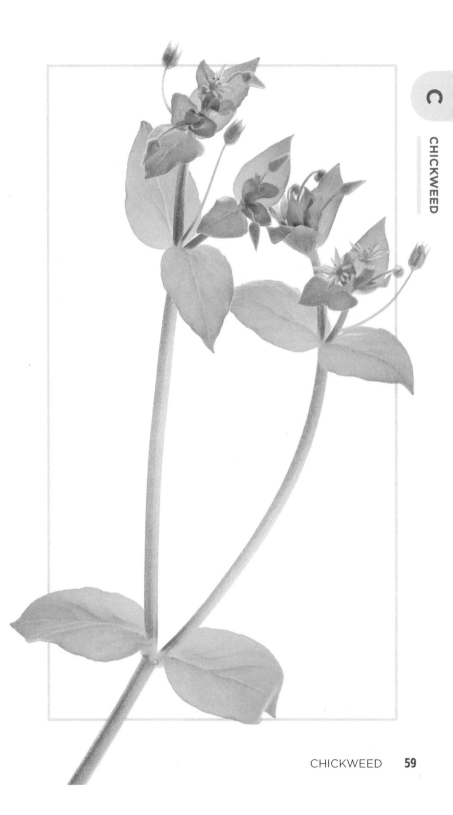

Cleavers

Cleavers emerges at the most convenient time, almost as if nature knows that we need its healing touch after a long winter. Most people regard these common yard "weeds" as a nuisance that appears in early spring. They are easily identified by their texture; cleavers plants are very sticky, and they'll stick to your skin, clothes, and even one another. What makes the plant useful is its ability to cleanse the lymphatic system, promote lymph flow, and aid in the elimination of toxins. During the winter months, our bodies can become quite stagnant. We spend more time indoors with little sunlight, we typically eat less healthily over the holidays, and our moods can become more depressed. As a result, our immune systems can become bogged down and make us feel sluggish and sickly. A tincture made with freshly harvested spring cleavers can help support the immune system, boost production of lymphocyte (a type of white blood cell), reduce swelling, and lower inflammation in the lymph glands so we can feel better. Instead of pulling and composting these common garden and yard weeds, consider collecting some to make the Lymph Support Cleavers Tincture.

Find the Cleavers remedy on page 154.

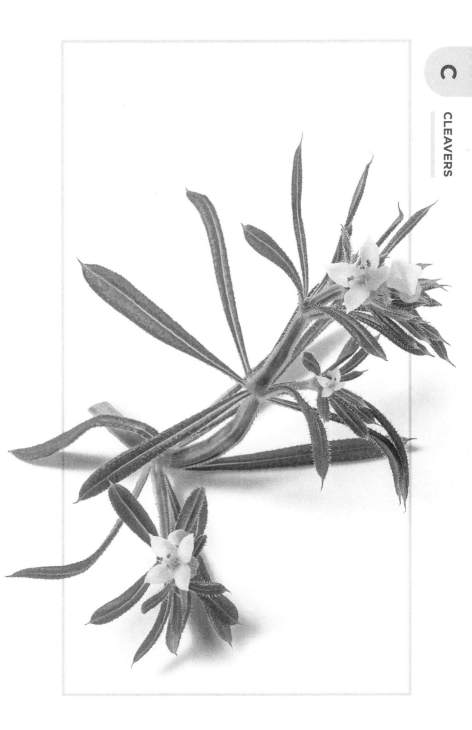

Comfrey

Comfrey isn't just a beautiful addition to an herb garden. It has been called "bone knit" for its ability to soothe and heal fractures, sprains, and other trauma. A few years back, I tripped on a rock and twisted my ankle very badly. It immediately started swelling, and I couldn't even stand up to get help. Luckily, I had my phone with me. A neighbor took me to the emergency room; I had a fracture, but nothing too serious. The pain and swelling were getting worse and worse, so when we got home, I had my husband go out and grab a giant comfrey leaf, and I applied it directly to the ankle with a wrap to hold it in place. Every 4 hours or so, I replaced the leaf with another. The swelling and pain were almost gone within 24 to 48 hours. Ever since, I make sure to always have comfrey in my garden. Though applying the leaf by itself is a really quick and easy method, you can make this salve to apply to sprains, fractures, and swollen areas to reduce swelling and pain.

Find the Comfrey remedy on pages 155–156.

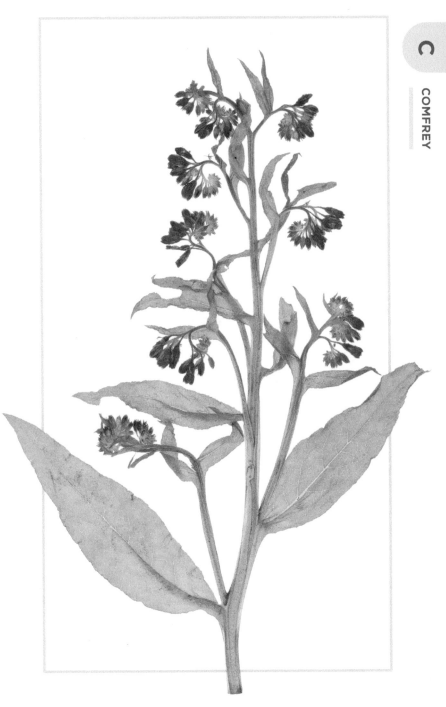

Cottonwood

There's a very old herbal remedy called "Balm of Gilead."
It takes its name from the plant of the same name that's
mentioned in the Bible, though no one knows what the
original really was. But the North American version is made
from the buds of the cottonwood, a common tree with
somewhat heart-shaped leaves that have serrated edges.
In the summer, you may notice a cottonwood tree by the
massive amounts of a cotton-like substance the male trees
produce. When you identify a cottonwood tree, visit it again
in the winter. That's when the trees produce resinous buds
full of medicinal goodness. (In some regions, this will be
in early spring). Just keep checking the tree and squish a
bud or two to see if your fingers become sticky with the
resin. This means its time to harvest. This resin has a unique,
camphorous aroma that is quite pleasant. It has been used
historically to treat areas of inflammation and pain. It can
be rubbed into painful, swollen areas to bring much-needed
relief. People have used this balm for arthritis, rheumatic
conditions, and anything else that causes pain and
inflammation.

Find the Cottonwood remedy on pages 157–158.

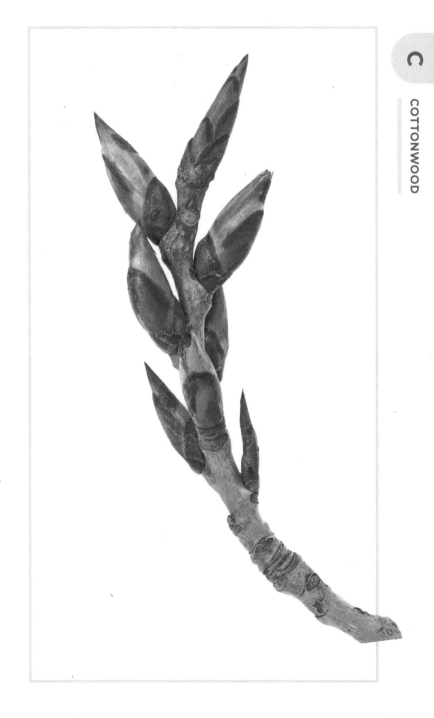

Dandelion

We all know this sunny yellow flower, but what many people don't realize is just how amazing and versatile it is! (If you don't look carefully, you might confuse it with the similar-looking cat's ear plant.) In fact, all parts of the dandelion plant have a purpose and a use. The flowers are edible and can be a tasty and colorful addition to a salad. You can also make dandelion fritters with them. The leaves are a rich and nutrient-dense source of vitamins and minerals. They can be eaten in a salad or stir-fry, or however you feel like preparing them. They are an herbal bitter, meaning they can aid in the digestion process for those who have gastrointestinal issues. However, it is the roots that are medicinally renowned; dandelion root gathered in fall of the first year of growth, or spring of the second year, is the most potent. Dandelion roots are a powerful tonic and diuretic. They can help cleanse and purify the body from the inside out, which can help support the liver, kidneys, and other detoxification organs. Because of its diuretic properties, dandelion root can support the urinary system to protect against urinary tract infections (UTIs) and other issues. If you feel sluggish, worn down, or like your body has a buildup of toxins, drink dandelion root tea to flush those out and feel your best. For those with skin issues like acne, dandelion root can help cleanse toxins that manifest on the skin. Glowing, healthy skin is within your reach!

Find the Dandelion remedy on page 159.

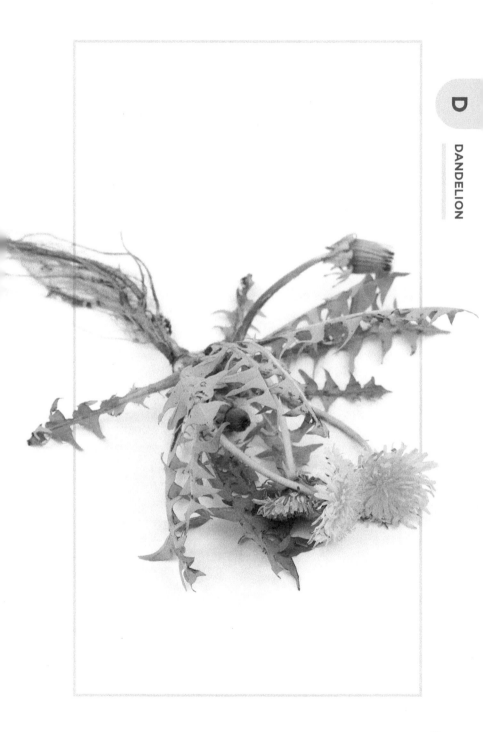

Echinacea (Purple Coneflower)

Standing tall and proud during the summer months, purple coneflower is a common sight along roadsides and in fields. This stately pollinator can grow up to 5 feet in height. Its bright purple-pink petals surround a prickly orange-and-black dome of seedheads. This plant is native to North America and was used extensively by some Indigenous peoples to cure a variety of infections, both viral and bacterial. There are several species of purple coneflower that grow throughout North America, with the most popular for medicinal use being *Echinacea purpurea*. Unlike some other plants, both the aerial parts of the plant and the roots are used in botanical remedies. Combining the different parts creates a powerful and synergistic remedy. Use discretion when harvesting this plant in the wild, as it is threatened in some areas. I grow it in my garden for this reason. Echinacea is very easy to grow: I threw some seeds out in early spring, and a year later I had a garden bed with plants up to my chest in height. They won't get very big the first year, but after that they will likely bloom to their full potential. I tend to dig up a few roots each fall but leave the rest to come back the next year. I harvest all aerial parts in the summer when the plant is in full bloom, using scissors or a sharp knife to make a clean cut on the stem.

Find the Echinacea remedy on page 160.

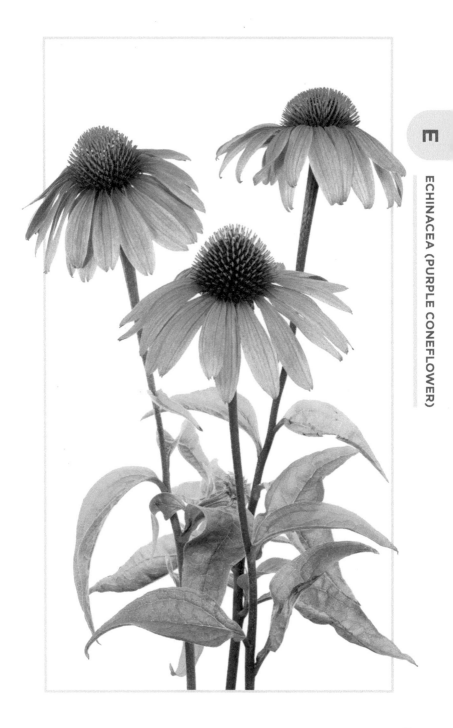

Elderberry

Where I live, elderberry bushes are everywhere and can easily be spotted in June due to the large umbels (umbrella-shaped clusters) full of white flowers. These flowers will eventually turn into tiny, dark berries in the fall. I prefer working with our native elderberry (*Sambucus canadensis*) here in the Midwest, but other species are just as good, such as *Sambucus nigra*. Elderberry has soared to popularity in recent years for its immune-boosting properties. It can stop a virus in its tracks if it is taken early. I have made many preparations with elderberry; after much trial and error, I've come to find that the traditional "elderberry syrup" is not as potent as the remedy in this book. Raw honey is a great and medicinal product on its own, but adding a large amount to your boiled elderberry juice, as many recipes call for, only serves to dilute the main and most antiviral ingredient in the preparation. I've made this elderberry remedy for people in my community during cold and flu season, and folks loved it so much that I accrue a large waiting list every year. The remedy is still tasty and sweet yet more concentrated, so you can kick a virus faster.

Find the Elderberry remedy on pages 161–162.

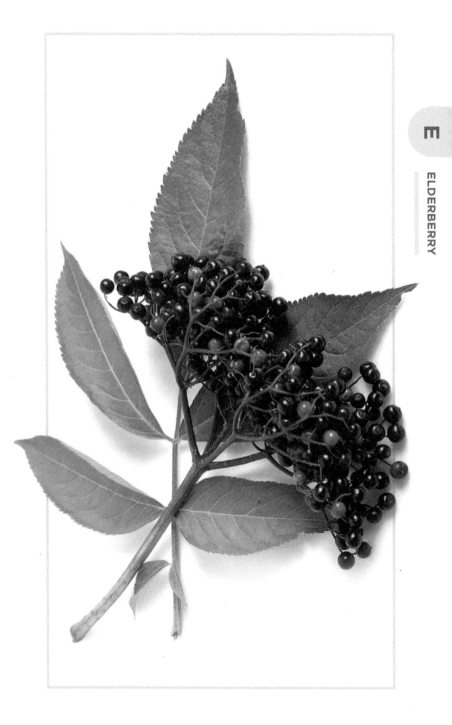

Fennel

In ancient Greece, it was believed that drinking a cup of fennel seed tea would give soldiers the strength and courage they needed for battle. All parts of the fennel plant have a highly aromatic, licorice-like scent. This herb has a long history of medicinal and culinary uses. Fennel is especially known for its digestive and gastrointestinal benefits. It helps relax gastrointestinal muscles to naturally relieve digestive complaints like bloating, gas, indigestion, and constipation. In addition, it may help relieve inflammation in the digestive tract and reduce spasms. All parts of the plant are used for food and medicine, but the seeds are most often used to make tea. Fennel has been studied for its effect on menopausal women and has been shown to reduce symptoms like insomnia, vaginal dryness, and hot flashes. Its hormone-balancing effects may also make it useful for premenstrual syndrome (PMS). The fact that it helps with bloating is a bonus, since many women who suffer from PMS and other menstrual issues complain of bloating also. Try a cup of fennel seed tea when you feel gassy, bloated, or need relief from digestive woes. And who knows—you may feel ready for a good battle afterward.

Find the Fennel remedy on page 163.

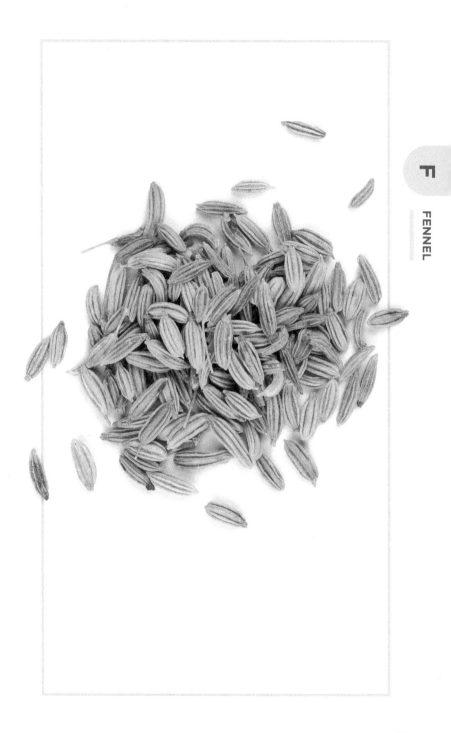

Goldenrod

Let's set the record straight about goldenrod once and for all: This plant is usually blamed for fall allergies because it happens to bloom around the same time as ragweed. But almost every time, ragweed is to blame for allergies, not goldenrod. In fact, goldenrod is pollinated by insects, and it's wind-pollinated plants (like ragweed) that are usually the culprits for allergies. This beautiful golden plant is a kind of harbinger for fall; when I see goldenrod, I know that autumn is right around the corner, and it makes my heart happy! It's full of antioxidants, having more than green tea. In addition, goldenrod possesses strong anti-inflammatory properties. Goldenrod is also diuretic, so it can help flush out toxins and excess water from the body. Its antimicrobial properties help kill bacteria in the digestive and urinary tracts. It is this combination of medicinal attributes that makes goldenrod so useful for treating urinary issues like UTIs and bladder infections. It can soothe an inflamed urinary tract and bladder as well as kill bacteria responsible for causing an infection. For best results, make a strong tea with this plant at the first sign of a UTI. Drink plenty of water to keep flushing out your system during this process. There are many types of goldenrod out there; I haven't found any to be unsuitable, but the most common for medical use is *Solidago canadensis*, probably because it's the most abundant.

Find the Goldenrod remedy on page 164.

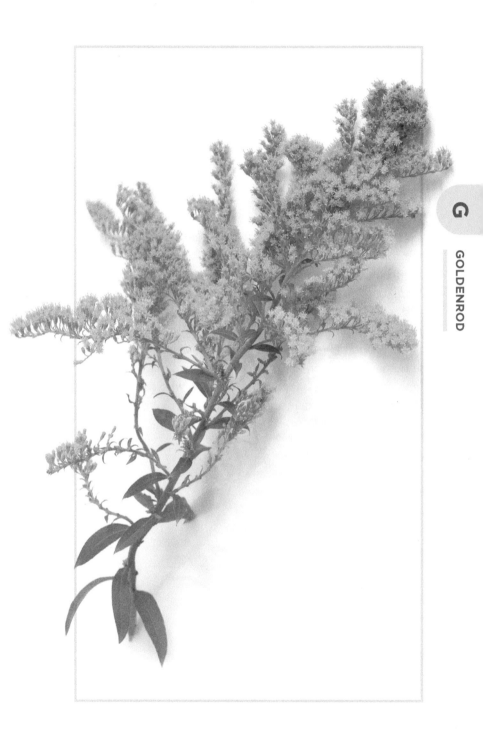

Hops

One summer, I went to visit my cousin and noticed green clusters hanging on plants at the woods' edge. Upon further inspection, I discovered that it was hops. This vining plant was growing all over the place, and the pale green clusters of flowers were hanging like grapes ripe for the picking. The hops plant has a rich history of use as a flavoring in beer, but it also possesses some interesting medicinal properties. The plant is sometimes called "lupulo," and it can be used for its sedative and nerve-calming properties. If you have trouble falling asleep or settling down in the evenings, a hops-based remedy might just be perfect to help quiet a distressed mind and bring stillness to a restless body. Another interesting tidbit about hops: The plant contains phytoestrogens that may mimic the way estrogen works in the human body. For this reason, the hops plant is used by menopausal and perimenopausal women who need help managing hormone balance, insomnia, and night sweats.

Find the Hops remedy on page 165.

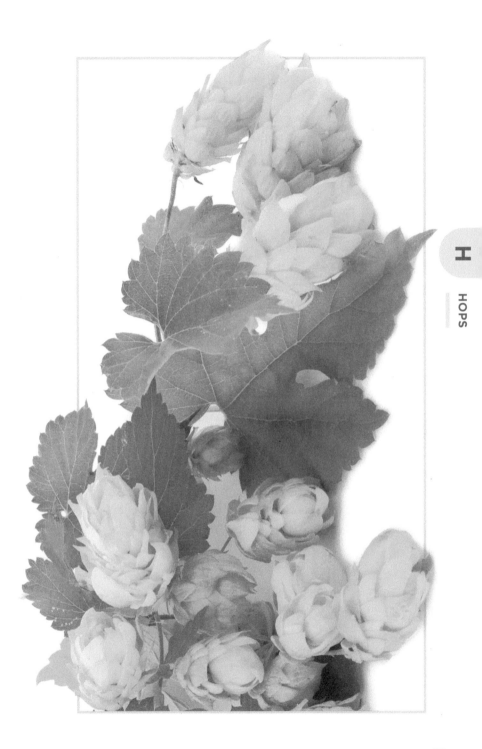

Japanese Honeysuckle

Perhaps you have deduced this already from the name, but this plant is definitely not native to North America. But it's here, and the invasive and aggressively spreading vine happens to have some extremely beneficial (and surprising) uses. Perhaps you already know that the flowers are medicinal and have astringent and skin-soothing properties, but did you know that the whole vining plant is highly antiviral? So why not make the most of this plant when you rip it out of your yard? I have a section of fence that is taken over by this plant; it can be really annoying because it encroaches upon my garden area. When I go outside in the summer to pull it out and keep it at bay, I harvest a basketful to make a tincture for treating viruses. There's no need to pick just the flowers; go ahead and rip that thing out, vine and all! All parts of the vine can be chopped and tinctured to make an extract that inhibits viral replication. Do not confuse this species (*Lonicera japonica*) with other invasive honeysuckle species, like bush honeysuckle. Bush honeysuckle is easy to tell from the vining honeysuckle because it grows like a woody shrub instead of a vine. There have been claims that this plant inhibits pregnancy, though clinical evidence is hard to find. Nevertheless, you may want to play it safe and avoid this plant if you're pregnant or trying to conceive.

Find the Japanese Honeysuckle remedy on page 166.

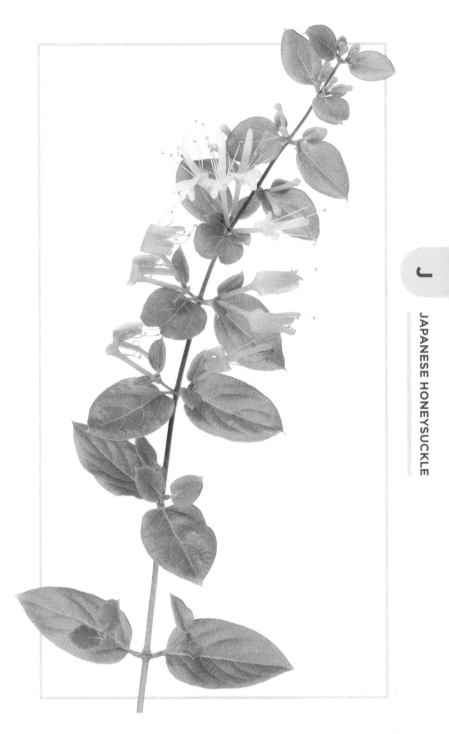

Juniper

Junipers are evergreen trees that produce little blue berries; there are many juniper species, but it's the common juniper, *Juniperus communis*, that we use for a wide array of medicinal remedies, which range from supporting urinary health and digestion to lowering blood sugar and easing insomnia. One of the most popular historical uses for juniper berries is as a flavoring in gin; they are still used today by many gin manufacturers. You can infuse these versatile berries in water to make tea to treat indigestion, insomnia, and UTIs. Juniper berries are very helpful when taken internally for a variety of complaints, and they're also great for skin issues. They can promote healthy skin due to their antioxidant content. Juniper berries are perfect for helping heal stubborn wounds and skin rashes as well. Add the fact that they are antimicrobial and antifungal, and you have a great reason to add these berries to your skincare routine. Since they come from evergreen trees, juniper berries can be harvested in the winter. They make the perfect winter remedy for dry skin and can also help soothe inflammation and tired, sore muscles.

Find the Juniper remedy on page 167.

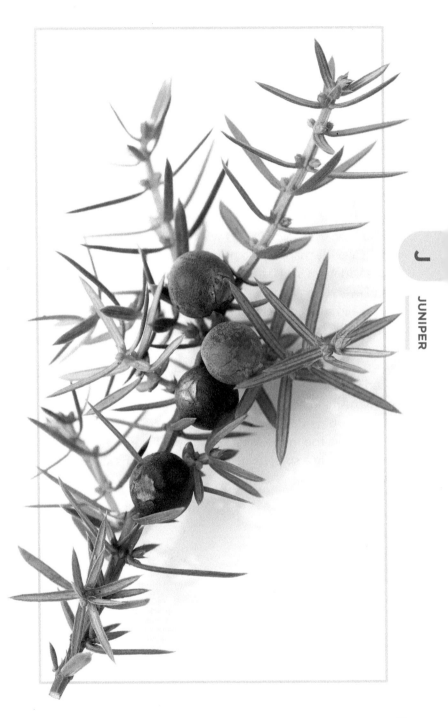

Lavender

In 1910, a French chemist by the name of René Maurice Gattefossé burned his hand in a perfumery lab. Fate intervened when in a frenzy (and probably a lot of pain) he dipped his hand in the nearest liquid he could find. It happened to be lavender essential oil. To his surprise, he noticed that his badly burned hand healed rather quickly—and with little scarring. He attributed this to the lavender and spent his days thereafter experimenting with it. He even used lavender on WWI soldiers in military hospitals. Lavender happens to be an especially nourishing plant for a variety of skin issues, ranging from burns to rashes (and everything in between). As if that isn't enough, it has also been studied for its ability to boost the mood and lower blood pressure. Lavender (meaning *Lavandula angustifolia*, or English lavender, one of over 40 lavender species) has a wonderfully herbaceous and floral aroma that has been used in perfumes for centuries. The aroma alone can calm the mind and body. This powerful plant is a must-have in any herb garden. It is easy to grow in containers and doesn't like too much water. One of my favorite ways to use this plant is in a spray to soothe skin conditions like burns, rashes, and minor lacerations.

Find the Lavender remedy on page 168.

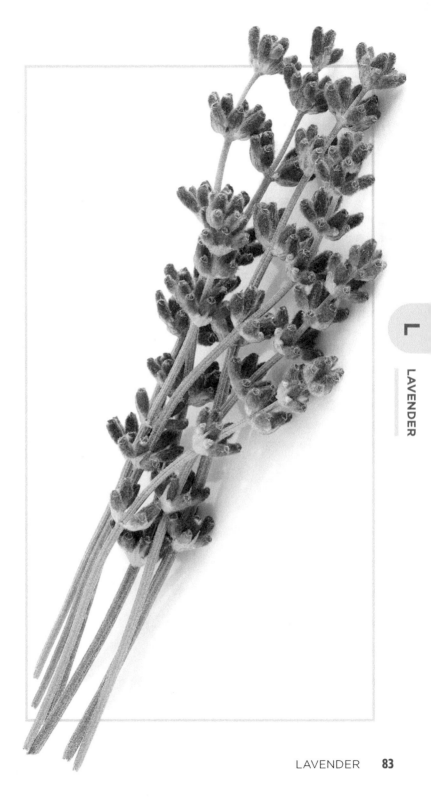

Lemon Balm

Lemon balm (also referred to as "Melissa") might be among the top contenders for plants anyone can grow. Even if you have a "black thumb," you'll find that lemon balm is forgiving and spreads quite fast. In fact, you'd better keep an eye on it, because in some areas lemon balm might escape cultivation and start its own colony. It spreads like a mint because it is a member of the mint family. I sowed some seeds in one of my raised beds a while back, and the plant somehow jumped out of the beds and is now growing in the yard. So when we mow, we are hit with a wonderful citrusy scent that honestly makes the boring task of mowing the grass more enjoyable. This uplifting plant's lovely lemony aroma makes for a very tasty and invigorating tea. It is also used in cooking for its lemony flavor. Lemon balm has several important medicinal properties. It can help heal viral lesions (like cold sores), nourish the digestive tract, and calm frazzled nerves. When you feel anxious or stressed, try lemon balm for some quick comfort.

Find the Lemon Balm remedy on page 169.

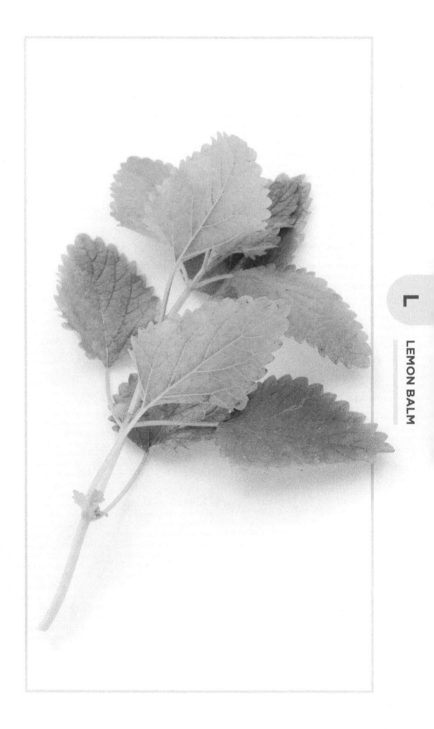

Marshmallow

When I was a child and heard about this plant, I couldn't believe that a plant was responsible for making my favorite campfire treat. Although most marshmallows on the market today are made differently (most use gelatin in some form), the roots of the marshmallow plant were once used to make the popular snack. This is because they are an excellent mucilage, meaning the plant forms a soothing coating that can cool inflammation, spasms, and other agitations. Marshmallow plant root will form a gel-like substance when infused in water (and this is how marshmallows were once made). I cannot live without this plant, because it helps coat my urinary tract to prevent interstitial cystitis flare-ups and the bladder spasms that come with this disease. For those who suffer from digestive disorders and ulcers, marshmallow root can coat the stomach, intestinal lining, and even the urinary tract to soothe inflammation and prevent spasms, pain, and discomfort. It is also great for those who are prone to UTIs, because it can coat the bladder and urinary tract with antimicrobial goodness to soothe inflammation and fight infection. Try the infusion recipe in this book to experience relief from digestive and urinary complaints.

Find the Marshmallow remedy on page 170.

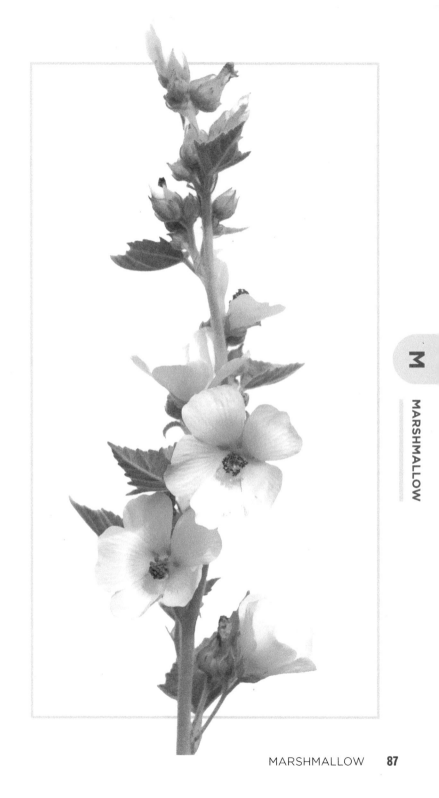

Mimosa

Nope, I'm not talking about the alcoholic beverage! Mimosa, Latin name *Albizia julibrissin*, has spread all over North America but is originally native to Asia. You may notice these trees along the highway during the late spring and summer months. They have an almost tropical appearance and produce these cute little pink flowers that resemble wispy puffballs. The flowers have an intoxicating smell that pollinators and hummingbirds love. We have one in our backyard, and it releases long, bean-like seedpods in the fall. These trees do spread easily, so we have to be careful not to let them take over and potentially harm our native tree species. In China, the mimosa tree is referred to as the "tree of happiness," and it has long been used to treat grief and sadness. For those looking for a gentle remedy for distress, sorrow, and heartache, mimosa may help you look on the bright side. I prepare a tincture from this plant to hand out in my community after losses and tragedies.

Find the Mimosa remedy on page 171.

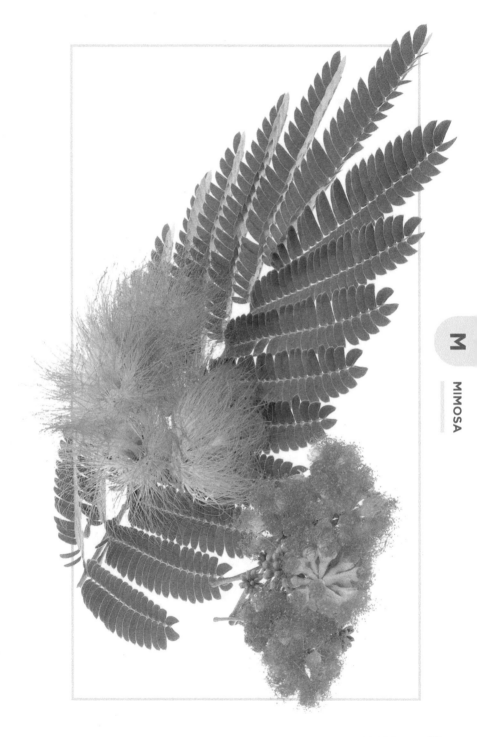

Motherwort

Motherhood isn't always easy, and for those times when you feel overwhelmed, frustrated, and overstimulated, motherwort can be a loyal plant friend. It has aided women for centuries. It is said that midwives used motherwort to help with stress during labor as well as to soothe anxiety in pregnant women. These uses are how the plant got its name. But motherwort's capabilities as a powerful yet gentle nervine aren't the only useful characteristics of this plant. It is also a wonderful cardiovascular protector. Motherwort can help heal and protect the heart and cardiovascular system by helping with high blood pressure issues (especially those brought on by stress) and easing irregular and rapid heartbeat brought on by stress and anxiety. I have found that motherwort is particularly useful for those needing help with sudden episodes of anxiety and stress that leave them feeling overwhelmed. When we allow ourselves to feel this way too often, it can be harmful to the cardiovascular system. Motherwort can bring balance back and help you feel more adept at handling life's stresses. Because of its ability to nourish the cardiovascular system, this member of the mint family was bestowed with the Latin name *Leonurus cardiaca*.

Find the Motherwort remedy on page 172.

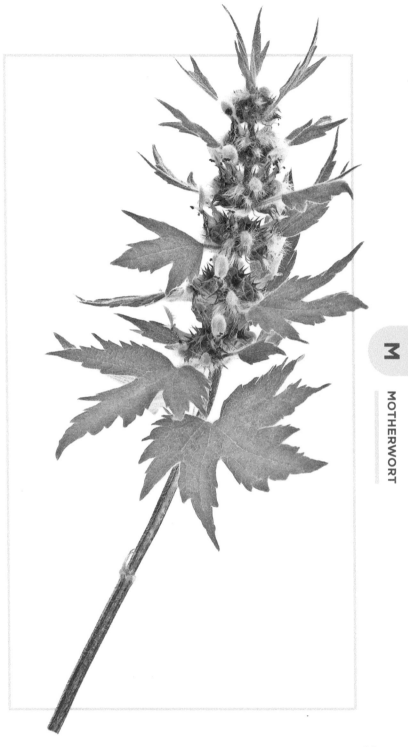

Mullein

This respiratory-nourishing plant has been used for centuries to break up congestion and mucus in the airways. The leaves are often used for this purpose. However, other parts of mullein boast additional unique attributes. For example, the yellow flowers that bloom along the tall stalk can be collected and infused in olive oil with some garlic to make a very effective ear infection remedy. The roots are analgesic as well (only the roots in the fall of the first year of growth or in the late spring of the second year) and have been used since ancient times to treat nerve and back pain. In fact, the Abenaki, Indigenous peoples from Canada and the United States, would make a necklace from the roots for their babies to wear when they were teething. Mullein shares a colorful and interesting history due to its versatility of uses. This tall plant starts out with fuzzy leaves in a basal rosette pattern. In its second year of growth, a stalk emerges that can get quite tall. Yellow flowers grow along the stalk. It prefers disturbed areas; for example, if you have bulldozing work on your property, you will likely see a few plants (or a whole forest of them) emerge a few months later.

Find the Mullein remedy on page 173.

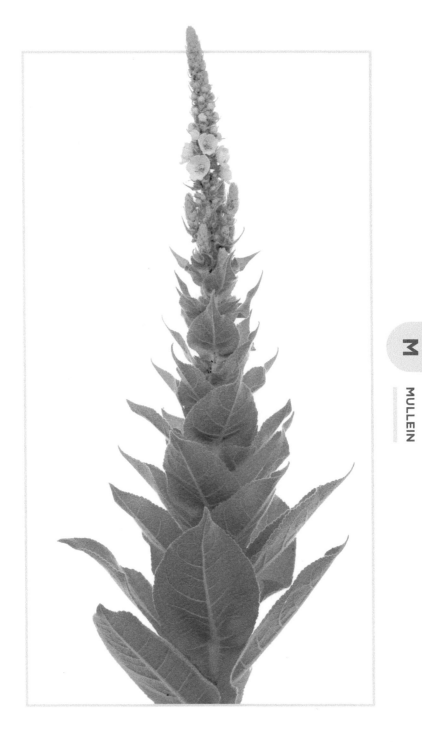

Oregano

Oregano is one of the most popular culinary and medicinal herbs for a reason! For starters, it is very easy to grow. I threw a few seeds in my garden one year, and now I have a hard time keeping the oregano from taking over. Native to the Mediterranean area, oregano tolerates dry conditions quite well and does best in full sun, although mine is doing great in a shady area of my garden. If you don't have room in your garden for this plant, it can be grown in containers just about anywhere. The best way to identify this herb is to smell it—the aroma of oregano is unmistakable! Also look for small and rounded leaves. My favorite thing about this plant is its strength. That strong smell is indicative of its strong antimicrobial, antibiotic, and antibacterial properties. I have so much oregano in my garden that I sometimes steam-distill it to make essential oil, but the oil is really, really potent. It can burn the skin if it isn't diluted. You don't have to worry about burning your skin with this plant, though, if you make an oil infusion, which isn't as concentrated as an essential oil. That means it is safer to massage into the skin, so you can use it when you need it with no worries. Learn to make your own potent oregano oil infusion later in this book.

Find the Oregano remedy on pages 174–175.

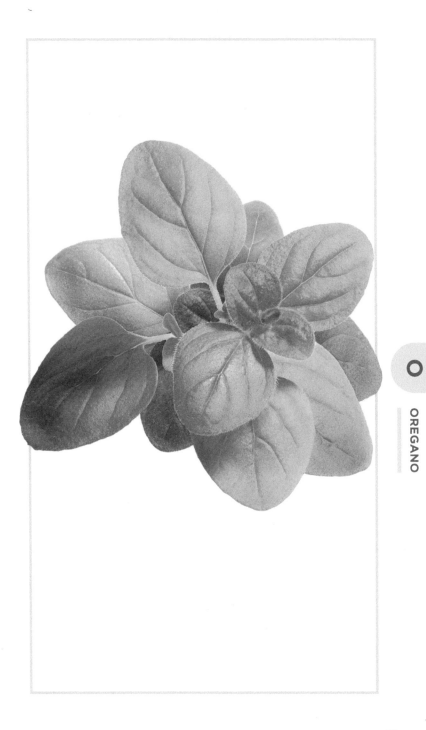

Passionflower

This plant, hands down, has the most beautiful flower I have ever laid eyes on. Passionflower is a vine that's really easy to grow from starters. So to add a pop of color and beauty to your deck or yard, I highly recommend passionflower. The flower is so intricate and so mesmerizing! It comes in a variety of shades, but the most common (*Passiflora incarnata*) is white and purple. After the flowers have gone, the plant bears an edible, kiwi-size fruit called "passionfruit." It is a plant steeped in legend and has a rich history. It is said that monks used the flower to teach others about Christ; a central stamen (shaped somewhat like an X) was said to represent the cross, and other parts represented apostles, and so forth. Passionflower is also a great nervine that can help with anxiety and everyday stresses that leave you feeling mentally fatigued. I tincture the aerial parts of this plant for a quick remedy that can reverse the effects of frayed nerves. In addition to sedative and nerve-soothing effects, passionflower is antispasmodic, making it helpful for conditions like restless legs syndrome.

Find the Passionflower remedy on page 176.

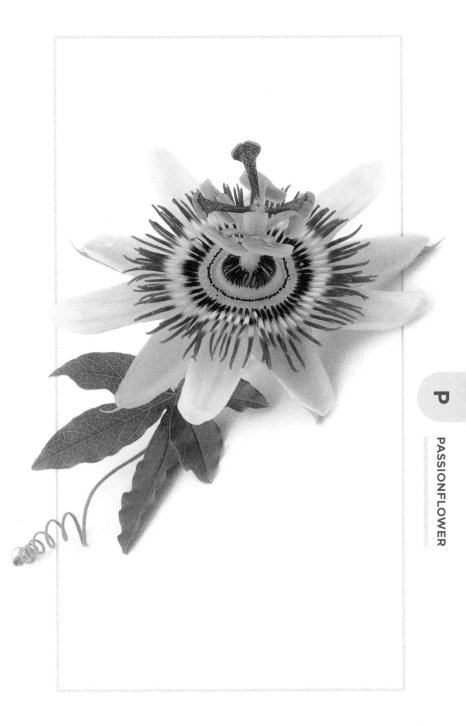

Peppermint

If you're looking for a medicinal plant that's ridiculously easy to grow, let me introduce you to peppermint. This common culinary and medicinal herb spreads quickly via a system of runners, so plant it in a contained area! I currently have a neglected, broken pot sitting outside on my front porch. A neighbor had given it to me full of peppermint a few years ago. I only water it when I remember, it doesn't get much sun, and the poor pot has seen better days. Yet every year, even after a long and frigid winter, peppermint continues to spring up and thrive throughout the spring and summer months. In addition to its stress-free maintenance, peppermint boasts several important medicinal properties. It can help ease digestive upset and prevent spasms in the intestinal tract. It's great for issues like gas, bloating, and nausea as well. Topically, peppermint tea (cooled in the refrigerator) can make a soothing and refreshing sunburn spray. Its invigorating scent can energize and motivate. Another popular use for this plant is relief from headaches caused by migraines or tension. Most bugs hate the smell of peppermint, so it is commonly used in natural bug-repellant remedies. Try planting it around your house to deter creepy crawlies. All these uses make peppermint a versatile must-have in any herb garden.

Find the Peppermint remedy on page 177.

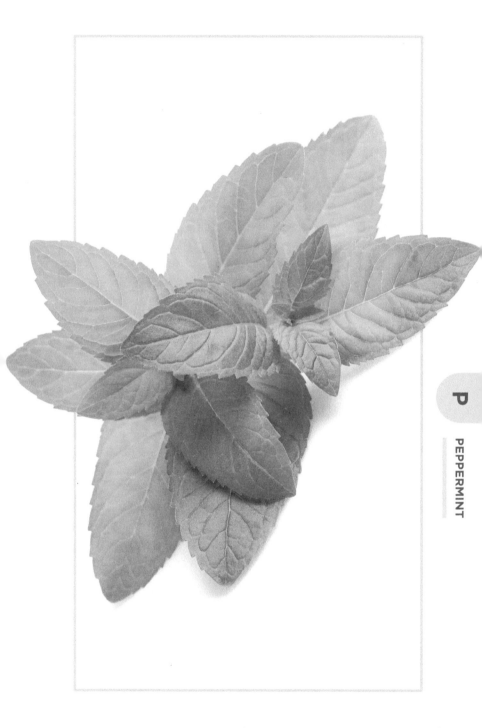

Pine

Not only are pine trees a common sight throughout most of North America, but they also hold great value to herbalists because they provide several kinds of plant medicine. First, the needles are a great source of vitamins A and C. Long ago, sailors used to drink pine needle tea to treat scurvy. They can provide the body with more than four times the amount of vitamin C than a glass of orange juice provides. Try infusing 2 teaspoons of chopped pine needles into a cup of hot water to make your own tea for immune health. Another medicinal part of the pine tree is the sap. Pine sap has long been used to treat a variety of respiratory issues, as well as rheumatic diseases and stomach ulcers. It has also been used in emergencies to bandage wounds naturally, and for drawing poison out of wounds. My favorite species of pine to use medicinally is the eastern white pine. The sap from this tree is naturally antibacterial, and its strong medicinal and aromatic qualities help open up the airways for those with bronchitis, coughs, and other respiratory complaints. We once had to chop off a few small branches on our pine tree to make room for a chicken coop in our yard. When we did this, the areas where the branches were removed began to ooze a resinous sap. I would go out once or twice daily and collect this sap until I had enough to make the powerful remedy on page 178. You are going to love the smell as well as what it can do for coughs, colds, and respiratory issues! Simply massage a small amount of this into the chest as needed.

Find the Pine remedy on pages 178–179.

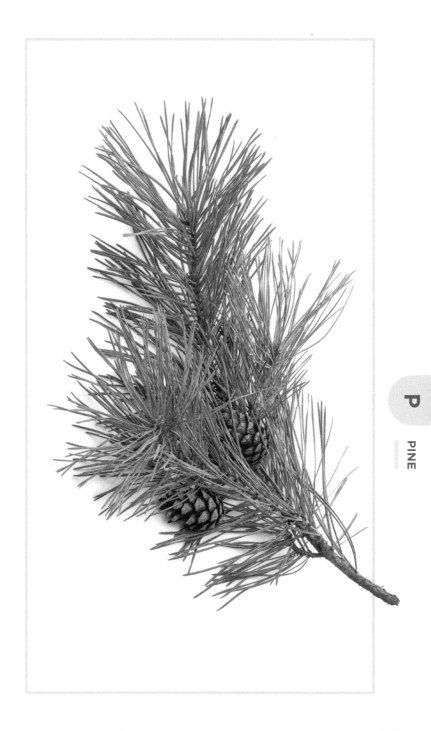

Pineapple Weed

This surprising "weed" holds a fun secret: It smells like pineapple! If you look closely at the plant, it may look suspiciously familiar. This is because it looks a lot like chamomile. The only notable difference between this plant and chamomile is that pineapple weed lacks the white petals chamomile has. These two plants are related and are both members of the genus *Matricaria*. This explains why they have such similar appearances and medicinal properties. In fact, pineapple weed can be used in the same way you would use chamomile. It makes an extremely tasty tea to calm frazzled nerves, soothe the mind, and even help you get the sleep you need. Its antispasmodic properties also make it useful for a cough or muscle spasms. The best thing about pineapple weed is you don't have to grow it. It tends to pop up in rocky, sandy areas in the spring and summer months, just waiting to be harvested. I found an endless supply near my sons' ballfield when I took them to practice one day. Once you first identify it, you will likely start seeing it everywhere. Softly rub the petalless yellow tops of the plant and take a whiff of that pineapple-packed aroma!

Find the Pineapple Weed remedy on page 180.

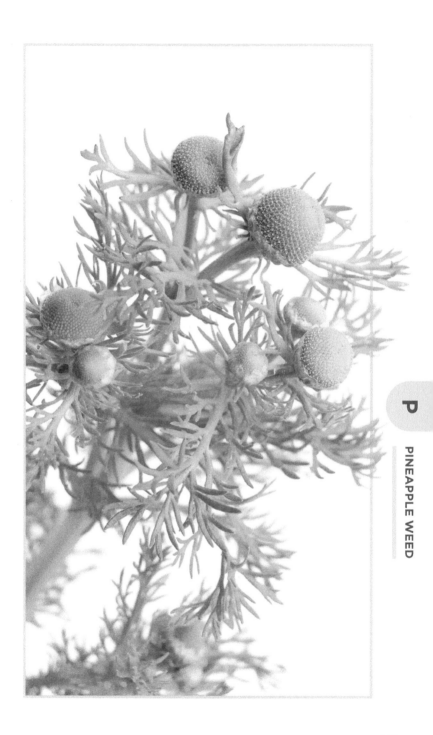

Plantain

Next to dandelion, broadleaf plantain (*Plantago major*) may be one of the most commonly found medicinal plants. It is literally all over the place. You can find it in yards, growing out of sidewalk cracks—it even grows out of my gravel driveway. Look for green, egg-shaped leaves growing in a rosette pattern (a circular arrangement of leaves). Leafless stalks emerge from the center of the leaves and are brown on top. Although many consider this plant to be a weed, it is surprisingly useful and may be one of my favorite medicinal herbs due to the fact that it can treat so many conditions. Plantain is always there when we need it; I can usually find it all year long, even in the winter months. The leaves possess natural antibacterial and anti-inflammatory properties. They are also mucilage, so they can be infused in hot water to make a tea for coating a sore throat and calming a hacking cough. Plantain tea is also antispasmodic and can quiet painful uterine cramps. It is great for skin; it can treat wounds, bruises, rashes, and other skin conditions. I have witnessed it pull splinters from the skin when crushed and applied topically. It can be infused in a carrier oil to make a soothing treatment for rashes, bug bites and stings, and inflammatory skin conditions. But I like to keep it simple and use the fresh leaves since they are so abundant.

Find the Plantain remedy on page 181.

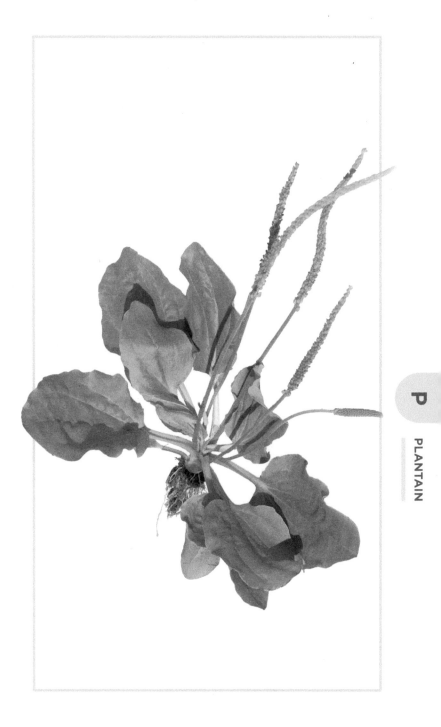

Purple Deadnettle

In the early spring months, you may notice tiny pink-purple flowering plants taking over your yard. These little members of the mint family are called "purple deadnettle" because the leaves turn a dark purple color closer to the top of the plant. This plant often grows with another similar member of the mint family called "henbit." Henbit can be distinguished from deadnettle by the leaves, which are smaller and a different shape than deadnettle (deadnettle leaves are toothed and come to a point). Both henbit and deadnettle are edible, so it isn't dangerous if you make an identification error with these two plants. They both have square stems and little pink, somewhat tubular flowers. Purple deadnettle contains flavonoids that help suppress histamine production in the body. This makes them especially useful in a tincture for seasonal allergies. You can tincture them in the spring for this purpose.

Find the Purple Deadnettle remedy on page 182.

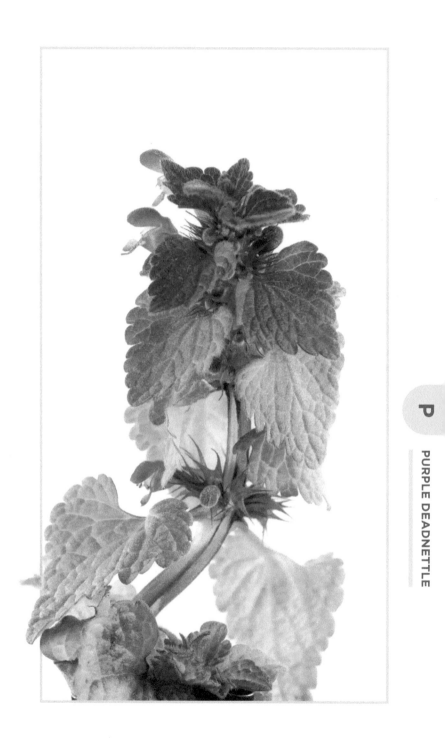

Red Clover

This clover is actually pink, which leads to a lot of confusion about the plant. And there is another species of clover that is red, called "crimson clover"—but the one we're focused on here is a lovely pink clover that just so happens to go by the common name "red clover." I don't make up the common names, but I apologize for the confusion nonetheless. The Latin name for this species of clover is *Trifolium pratense*. This plant is very common in North America and can be seen growing in the summer months in fields and along roadsides (but remember, never harvest any plant from the side of the road). It boasts several uses, including treating respiratory issues like asthma and whooping cough, and soothing skin irritations like psoriasis and eczema. Red clover contains phytoestrogens that act like human estrogen when they are introduced into the body. This makes it a promising remedy for menopausal and postmenopausal women. When estrogen levels are reduced during menopause, this can lead to bone loss and hormonal fluctuations that cause a variety of issues. Red clover can help balance estrogen levels to reduce hot flashes, bone loss, brittle hair and nails, night sweats, and even high cholesterol. It has diuretic properties, too, making it helpful for flushing excess water and waste out of the body. For this reason, it has also been used to help with urinary issues.

Find the Red Clover remedy on page 183.

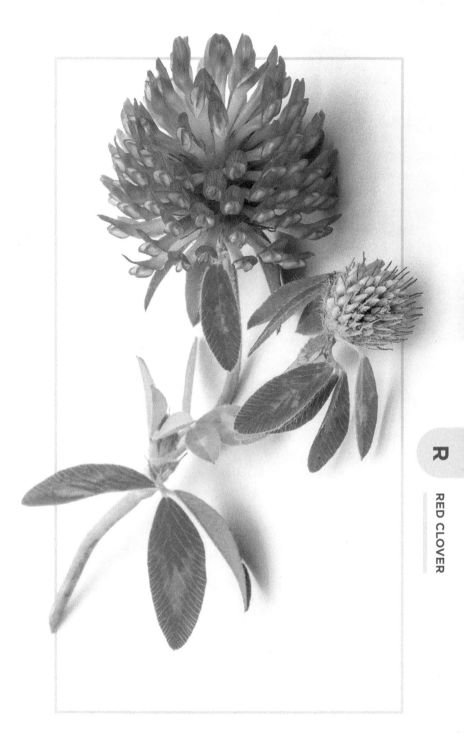

Red Raspberry Leaf

These vines practically take over the woods' edge on our farm. They can spread quickly if left unchecked! One way I distinguish red raspberry from other berry vines is the leaves: They are toothed around the edges and are often in groups of three. The underside is the giveaway, with a much lighter shade of green, almost white-green. Red raspberry leaves are a great source of nourishment, as they contain antioxidants, vitamins B and C, potassium, magnesium, zinc, phosphorus, and iron. Their nutrition content is only one part of their value, though. The other part lies in the fact that the leaves are a wonderful uterine tonic. There are some reports that red raspberry leaf stimulates uterine contractions; though this has not been proven, the plant has been used by pregnant women for centuries. Because it tones the uterus, red raspberry leaf is thought to help with easing and assisting childbirth as well as postpartum recovery. (Remember, if you're pregnant, talk to your doctor before using any herbal remedy.) It may even be a helpful remedy for women suffering from uterine fibroids, uterine prolapse, and heavy menstrual periods. That's because it's thought to help strengthen muscles around the pelvis to help with menstrual issues like cramping. Red raspberry leaf is a woman's friend indeed.

Find the Red Raspberry Leaf remedy on page 184.

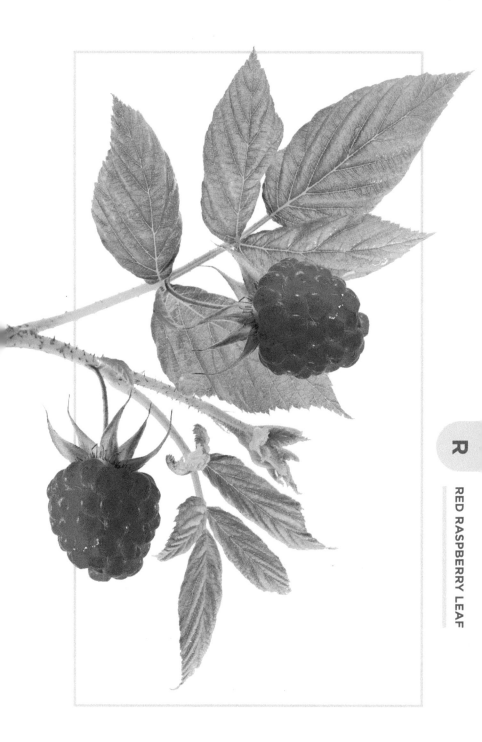

Rosemary

You can do a lot more with rosemary than flavor dishes (although it does have a wonderful flavor). In research studies, this popular culinary herb has been found to be as effective as Rogaine (a pharmaceutical hair loss treatment) for hair loss. It works by helping promote circulation on the scalp to nourish hair follicles and stimulate growth. Speaking of circulation, rosemary can also be used on other areas of the body to aid in blood circulation. For example, if you have circulation issues, you can infuse it into a carrier oil and then massage it into the legs. You can even infuse it into a cup of hot water to make a tea that promotes cardiovascular health and circulation. After losing a lot of hair (postpartum hair loss), I found rosemary to be especially effective for helping hair grow back and preventing more hair loss. My own personal success using rosemary for hair loss prompted me to include this amazing hair growth recipe.

Find the Rosemary remedy on pages 185–186.

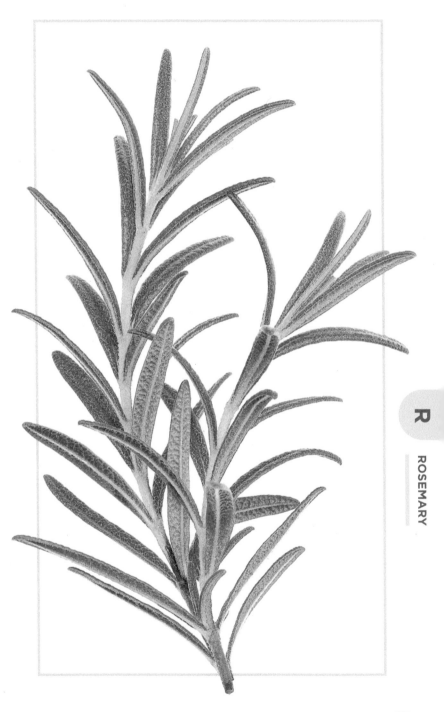

Self-Heal

Self-heal is also referred to as "heal-all." It comes by these titles honestly, because this little plant can treat a wide range of ailments. It has been used historically to treat wounds, rashes, infections, inflammatory conditions, fevers, gastrointestinal issues, and even viruses. One of its specialties is targeting the virus responsible for fever blisters. Self-heal can be taken internally (such as by infusing it in water to make tea) or applied externally to treat a variety of skin issues. It is a common sight in yards across North America during early summer months. Look closely and you are likely to see its purple, two-lipped petals appearing in clusters near the top of the plant. Self-heal's leaves grow in pairs along a square stem. When you find one, you will likely find many more, as this plant spreads quite rapidly via underground stems called "rhizomes."

Find the Self-Heal remedy on pages 187–188.

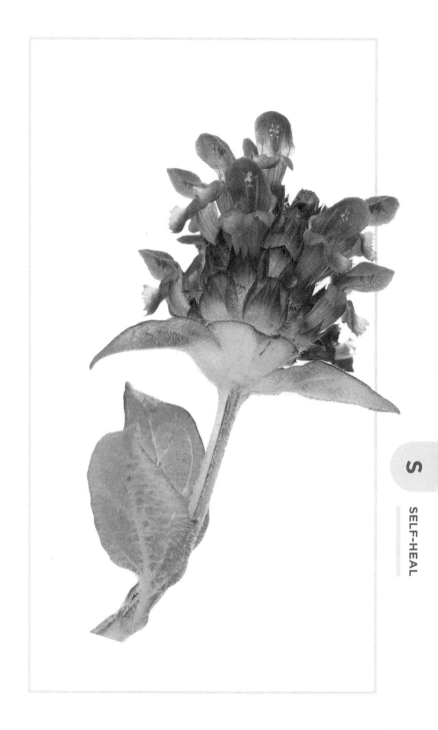

Skullcap

I was driving around my farm one day when I noticed some unusually shaped purple flowers. Upon closer inspection, I realized it was skullcap, *Scutellaria lateriflora*. This plant is native to North America and can be found growing at the woods' edge or in fields during the summer months. The unusual hooded violet flowers that grow up the top of the stem may be the reason for the plant's common name. Skullcap has also been called "mad dog skullcap," because it was historically used to treat "madness," or serious mental health conditions. It is a great nervine remedy, meaning it can calm the nerves for those feeling more than a little over-whelmed. In today's fast-paced society, it doesn't take much for one to feel in need of a mental break. If you need to chill out and calm down, run yourself a warm bath, grab a good book, and take a little of the tincture on page 189 to unwind.

Find the Skullcap remedy on page 189.

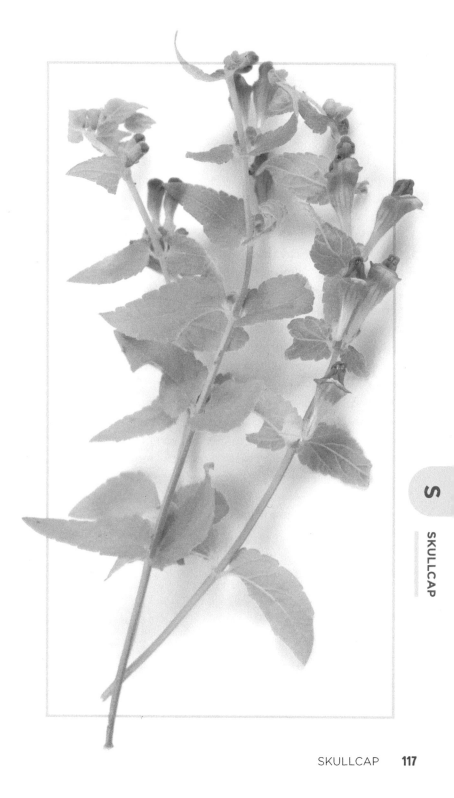

St. John's Wort

Summer solstice, the longest day of the year, occurs in mid-June. It is around this time of year when you may come across this little ray of sunshine, which fittingly blooms during the longest periods of daylight. The bright yellow flowers of St. John's wort are strong reminders of the joy and sunshine this plant can bring to people. St. John's Wort has long been used to treat mild to moderate depression and seasonal affective disorder (SAD). It acts on the nerves to bring peace, calm, and positivity. Because of these soothing nervine properties, this plant can also be used to treat nerve pain issues like sciatica. And it also possesses antiviral properties, so it can be used to treat cold sores and viral rashes. Look for bright yellow flowers that stain your fingers magenta when you rub the petals. This red tint inside the flowers is due to a compound called "hypericin," which is also the plant's primary medicinal compound. Leaves are lobed and tend to get bigger near the bottom of the plant. When you hold the leaf up to the sun, you may see tiny clear spots, or pores. To create a powerful remedy, it is best to use freshly harvested flowers. If you are on any medications, do your research before using this herb, as it can interact with some medicines.

Find the St. John's Wort remedy on page 190.

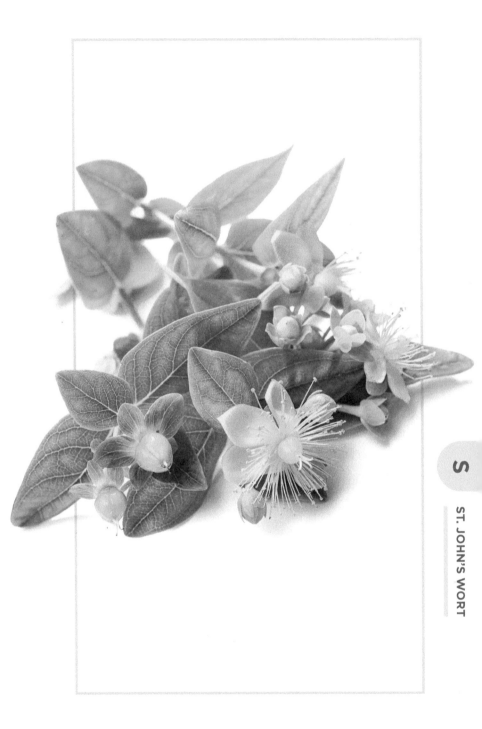

Stinging Nettle

Stinging nettle comes by its name honestly! If you happen to brush up against this common "weed," you'll definitely feel it. For this reason, it is advisable to wear gloves when harvesting this plant. Those tiny stinging hairs on its leaves and stem can cause skin reactions, but they are completely disarmed when the plant is harvested and dried thoroughly. They're also deactivated if you process the fresh plant into a tea, tincture, or any other medicinal preparation. For centuries, people used this plant to help with arthritis and related conditions by slapping it directly against arthritic joints—ouch! Thankfully, one doesn't have to do this to reap its benefits. Stinging nettle is diuretic, meaning it can help the body flush out excess water and impurities. For this reason, it is used as a remedy for urinary health. This plant also contains flavonoids that help reduce histamines in the body. In short, stinging nettle is very useful in a tea for allergies! It is also packed full of health-giving vitamins, minerals, and flavonoids. A remedy with stinging nettle is sure to provide the body with the nutrients needed for more rapid recovery from surgery as well as postpartum trauma or sickness.

Find the Stinging Nettle remedy on page 191.

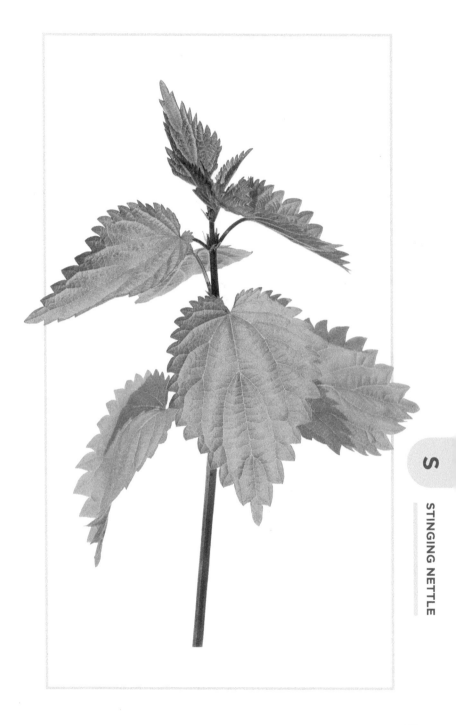

Sweet Gum

I'll be the first to admit that this tree can be a nuisance. If you are familiar with the sweet gum tree, you know that it produces spiky seed balls that cover the ground around the tree in the fall. You definitely don't want to be walking around barefoot in a yard where this tree is growing. I happen to have one right off my front porch, so trust me on that. But imagine my delight when I found out a secret about these seedpods: They contain a compound that is used to make a popular influenza drug called Tamiflu. This compound is called "shikimic acid." Both unripe sweet gum seed balls and pine needles contain this valuable compound. Please note that sweet gum will not act exactly like Tamiflu in the body, because the latter has been heavily altered in a lab to create the final product. However, I have personally had much success using sweet gum in a tincture alongside honeysuckle and/or elderberry to fight viruses like influenza.

Find the Sweet Gum remedy on page 192.

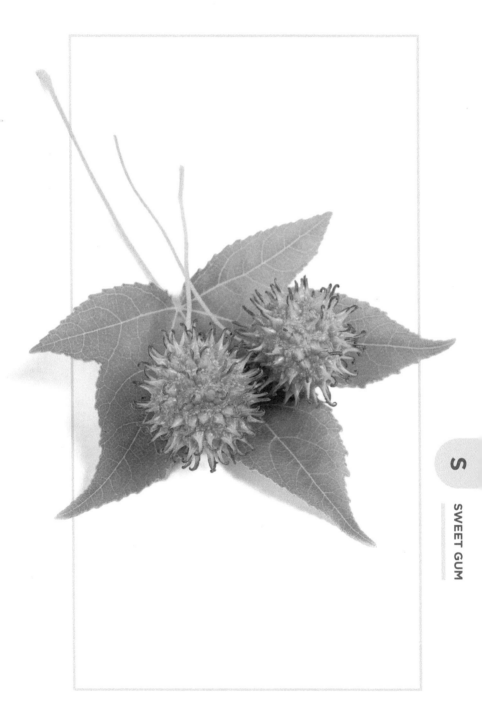

Sweet Wormwood

This plant is near and dear to my heart. It grows all over my farm in the summer months, and this past year it was still flourishing in late fall. It has a distinctive sweet scent that separates it from other *Artemisia* species. It can get quite tall and has highly divided leaves. This is a good time to let you know that this particular species, *Artemisia annua*, is a different plant from plain old "wormwood," *Artemisia absinthium*. We're talking about sweet wormwood here, or "sweet Annie," as it is sometimes called. Emerging research over the past two years has shown this plant to be effective at fighting off viruses. It works best in tincture form for this purpose. In addition to its ability to potentially interfere with viral replication, sweet wormwood is also antiparasitic, antimalarial, antimutagenic, and has been studied for its ability to induce apoptosis (cell death) in breast cancer cells. Do not take more than directed, as this remedy can cause diarrhea if it is misused.

Find the Sweet Wormwood remedy on page 193.

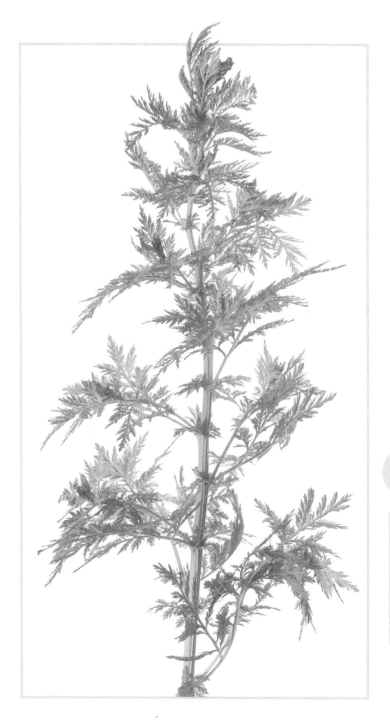

Valerian

This herbal version of the sandman may be just what you need if you have trouble falling asleep and/or staying asleep through the night. Valerian is an interesting flowering plant that can get pretty tall under the right conditions. The leaves are soft, dark green, and toothed around the edges. The most distinguishing feature of the plant isn't its appearance, though; it is the roots. When you dig these up, you will notice a very particular smell. Some say it smells like dirty socks, sweat, or dirty feet. Don't let these descriptions turn you off this remedy! Valerian has a lot to offer. Valerian roots contain compounds that act on the central nervous system as a sort of mild depressant. This is good for people who can't seem to calm down and fall asleep at night. Since it acts on the nerves, valerian also helps relieve pain, nerve spasms, anxiety, and depression. Valerian makes a superior alternative to products like melatonin supplements, which contain synthetic ingredients and may deplete the body's own ability to create melatonin itself (after years of repeated use). Try establishing a bedtime routine a few hours before bed, turning off ALL screens in the house—yes, that includes your phone—taking a warm bath, and having a cup of valerian root tea before you call it a night. Enjoy the restful sleep that ensues.

Find the Valerian remedy on page 194.

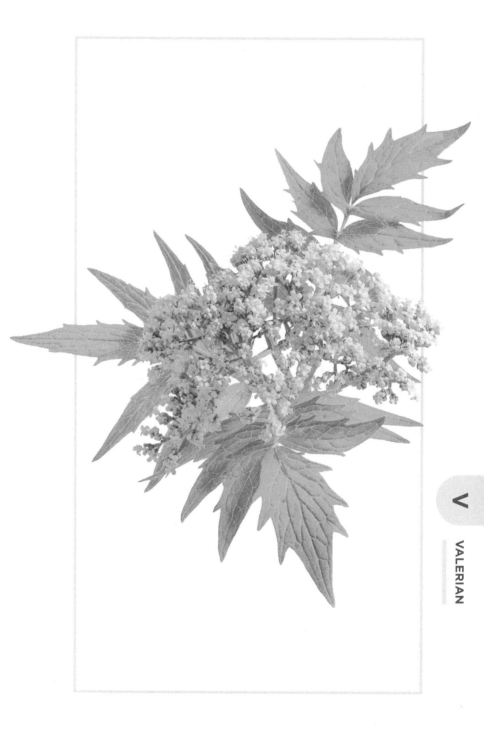

Violet

What a welcome spring sight! Violets usually start popping up on our farm in late March. There are many species of violets, but *Viola sororia* is our favorite for medicinal preparations. These violets have dark green, heart-shaped leaves and deep purple flowers that droop from the top of a stem. The flowers and leaves are edible. We harvest the flowers to use as a garnish for different dishes or to add a bit of vitamins A and C (as well as a pop of color) to a fresh spring salad. The leaves have historically been used in soups and stews as a thickener. Many people aren't aware that violet leaves are medicinal and mucilage (producing a gel-like substance that soothes and coats the throat, stomach, and intestines). For this reason, the leaves are useful in preparations for treating dry, hacking coughs, allergies, and sore throats. I prefer combining the leaves and flowers for a synergistic formulation that relieves sore throats and coughing.

Find the Violet remedy on page 195.

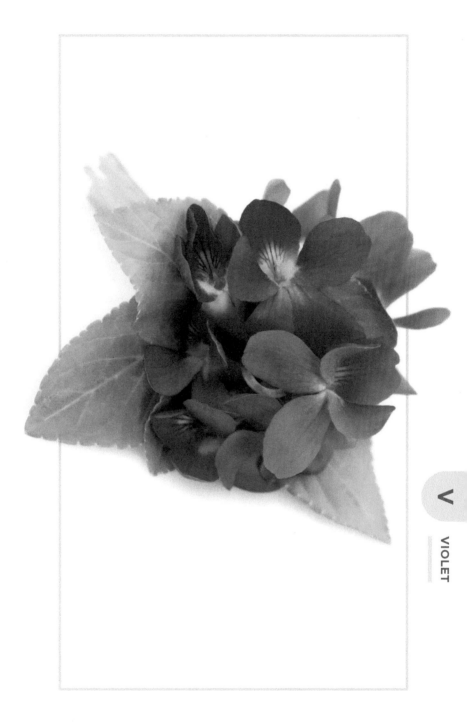

White Willow

The white willow tree happens to be a good source of a compound called "salicin." This compound is still used today to create what we know as "aspirin." The inner bark of the tree is anti-inflammatory, analgesic (pain-relieving), and febrifuge (it can lower fevers). Long before science discovered the presence of salicin, some Indigenous peoples were using white willow to treat pain, inflammation, and fevers. These trees are a common sight around North America, and they especially love wet areas. They have notoriously soft wood, so a good storm will result in several branches lying around the yard. This is the perfect time to harvest the bark. I grab fallen branches and then use a good knife to scrape them and collect the inner bark. Follow these directions to create a powerful tincture with white willow that I like to call "natural aspirin."

Find the White Willow remedy on page 196.

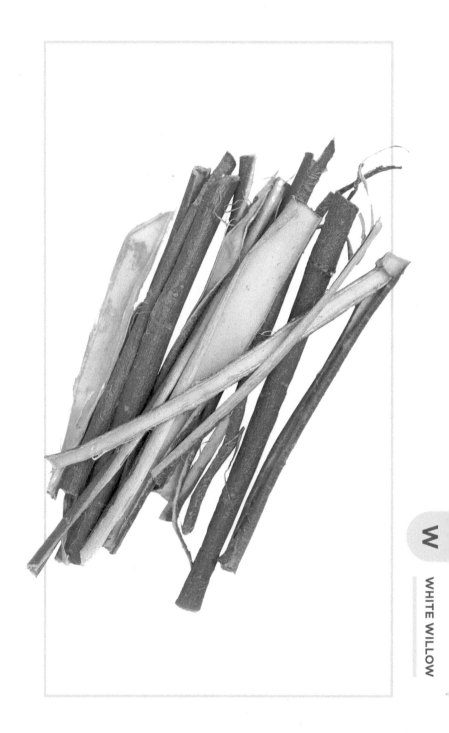

Wild Bergamot

Certain Indigenous peoples of North America made a tea from the leaves of the wild bergamot (*Monarda didyma*) called "Oswego tea." This tea was used to treat a variety of conditions, ranging from digestive issues to premenstrual syndrome (PMS). In the Midwest, where I live, a very closely related Monarda species (*Monarda fistulosa*) is used in much the same way. Monarda are sometimes referred to as "bee balm" or "wild bergamot" and are recognizable for their unique flower heads, which have tubular petals resembling wild hairs emerging from a head. The colors range from a violet hue to a deep magenta, depending on the species. The thymol content of this plant is likely where its medicinal uses come in. Thymol is a phytochemical known to be highly antimicrobial, antifungal, and antiviral. My whole house smells richly of a spicy yet herbaceous aroma when I make remedies with these flowers. I love to use the leaves and flowers to make a potent treatment for sore throats, coughs, and viruses.

Find the Wild Bergamot remedy on page 197.

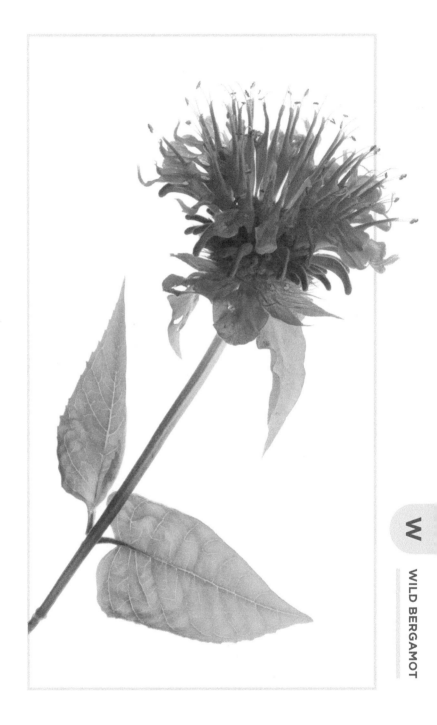

Wild Rose

There are many types of rose species that can be used medicinally, but the one I wish to discuss here is a sometimes invasive but naturalized species in most areas of North America. Wild rose (*Rosa rugosa*) can be found growing wild in fields and along roadsides in the summer months (but don't harvest roadside plants). The flower looks a bit different from a standard rose and has a pink hue with a yellow center. One of the things I like about this species is how common it is. It isn't hard to find a few when you go on a nature walk in the summer. Look for the bright pink flowers lying low to the ground (most don't get very tall). Another awesome attribute of this plant is its ability to produce larger fruit than many other rose species. The red fruits produced by roses in the fall are called "rose hips." They just so happen to be a great source of vitamin C. In fact, rose hips contain more vitamin C per tablespoon than citrus fruits. I like to collect these and throw a handful or two in my elderberry glycerite recipe (see page 161), or simply make a tincture with rose hips to take as a natural vitamin C supplement. It is also fun to combine both the flower and the rose hips to create a skin-softening and wrinkle-reducing facial serum. Rose petals are great for the skin and can reduce redness, inflammation, and acne. Rose hips can infuse the skin with a dose of vitamin C.

Find the Wild Rose remedy on page 198.

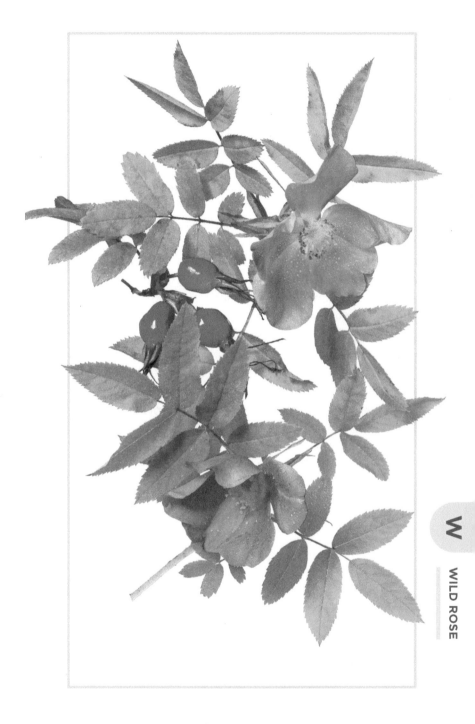

Witch Hazel

Witch hazel trees are an interesting and welcome sight when they bloom, for several reasons. One, they are known to bloom in the winter months, making a refreshing change of scenery amid a bleak and bare landscape. Two, the flowers themselves are quite peculiar, having ribbonlike yellow petals. The flowers, leaves, buds, bark, twigs, and new shoots of this tree are all worth collecting to create a healing and astringent formulation. Plants with astringent properties like this can soothe conditions like eczema, hemorrhoids, wounds, and acne. They can also support a healthier skin tone by eliminating redness, irritation, and inflammation. Along with toning the skin, witch hazel can tighten blood vessels, relax muscles, and even reduce the appearance of scars and stretch marks. You can create an infusion to add to a sitz bath for hemorrhoids, or even make a tea from witch hazel to drink for a sore throat or digestive issues. The possibilities are almost endless with this useful plant. Of all the uses for witch hazel, my favorite is for promoting healthy, clear skin.

Find the Witch Hazel remedy on page 199.

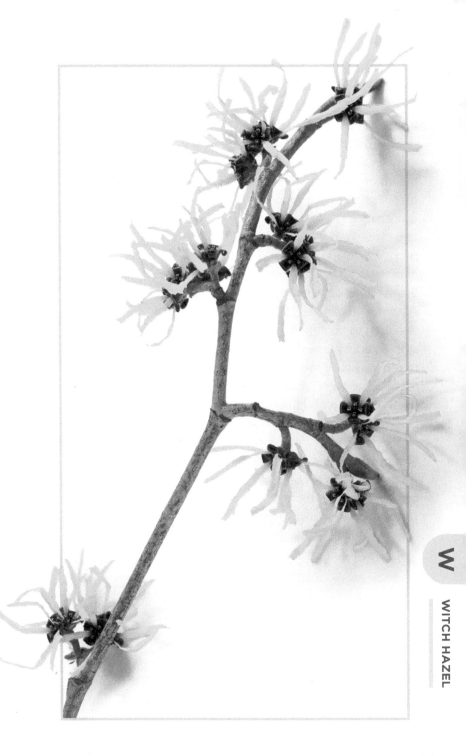

Yarrow

It is said that the Greek warrior Achilles used yarrow to help heal wounds on the battlefield. This legend gave yarrow its Latin name, *Achillea millefolium*. For centuries, yarrow has stood out as a great remedy to treat cuts, lacerations, bleeding, and other skin issues. Its styptic properties help reduce bleeding when the plant is poulticed (mashed up) and placed directly on a cut. In addition, its astringent properties help kill bacteria and reduce the chances of infection. Yarrow can also be taken internally (just infuse 1 to 2 teaspoons of the dried leaves and flowers in a cup of hot water for 10 minutes) to treat fevers, because it helps induce sweating to cool the body down. Just as yarrow helps stop bleeding for external wounds, it has also been used to reduce heavy menstrual bleeding. It doubles as a pain reliever and can reduce uterine spasms and cramping. This plant is widespread throughout most of North America and blooms from late spring to early fall. It can be detected by fernlike leaves that are bigger near the bottom of the plant. Cream-white flowers grow in clusters atop the plant. The whole plant has a medicinal, herbaceous aroma. Bugs rarely browse this plant because most are repelled by the scent of yarrow. For this reason, yarrow also makes a great natural tick, mosquito, and flea repellent.

Find the Yarrow remedy on page 200.

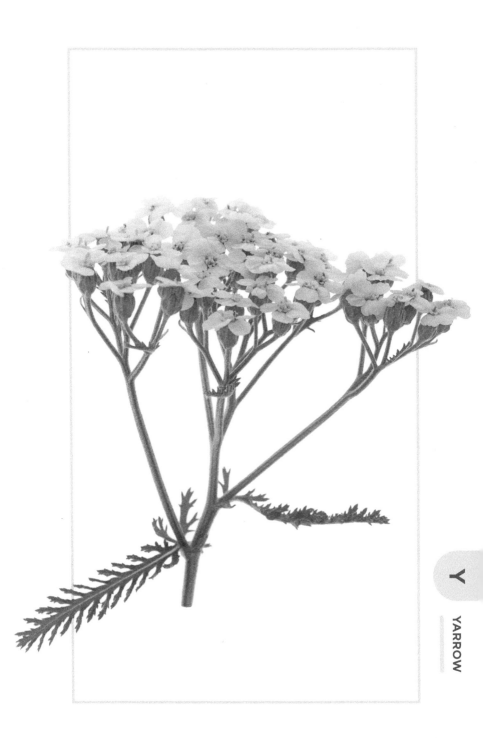

Yellow Dock

In the spring, we forage young dock leaves to sauté with other spring greens. The plant can be identified when it is young by looking at the leaves, which have curled edges. The plant is sometimes called "curly dock" for this reason. As it grows, it produces stalks full of seeds. When these seeds turn brown, they can be harvested to create a fiber-rich grain. The curled-edged leaves are a tasty edible that boasts medicinal properties. They can be poulticed and placed on bites, stings, and other skin traumas to bring down swelling. Yellow dock gets its name for its roots, which are a deep yellow hue. Some Indigenous peoples of North America used the roots of the first year of growth, harvested in the fall, to treat conditions ranging from yellow fever to rheumatism. The root has mild laxative effects and is a great source of iron (as are the leaves) and vitamins A and C. The iron content in this plant is helpful for those seeking a natural remedy for anemia. Yellow dock has tonic properties, and it belongs to a class of herbs known as "blood purifiers" (herbs that help remove toxins from the blood). As such, it has been used to treat diseases of the blood and skin. The root possesses astringent properties that can soothe upset bowels and digestive woes. It also helps with digestive upset by stimulating the production of bile to help the body break down fats and lipids more efficiently.

Find the Yellow Dock remedy on page 201.

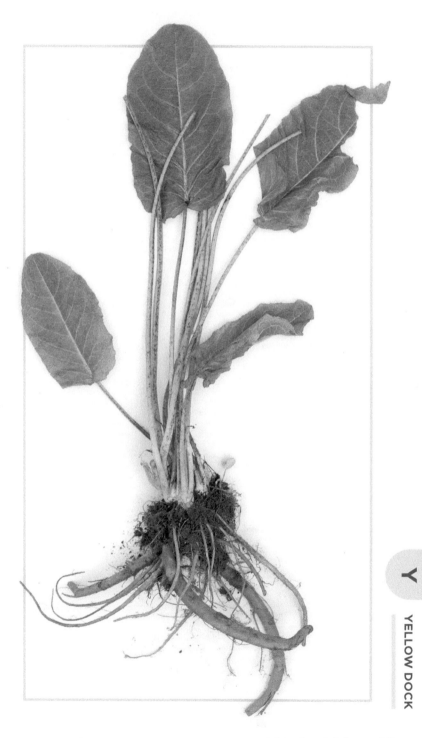

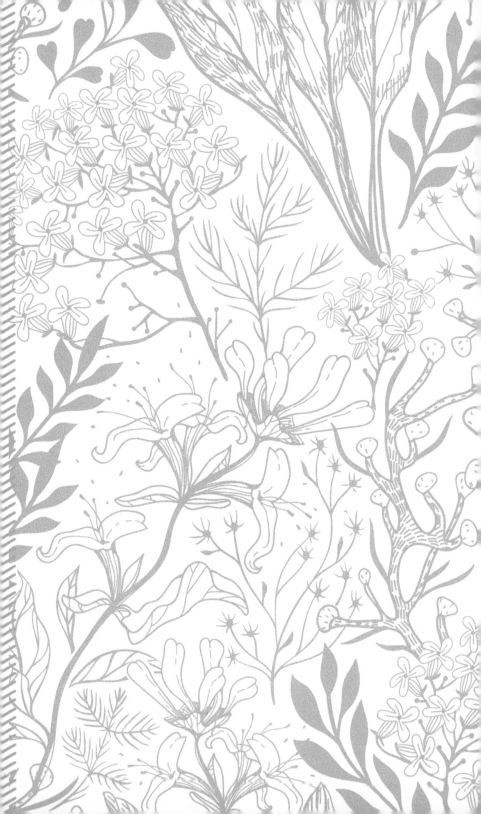

50
Essential
Remedies

Bowel-Soothing Agrimony Tea

Soothe irritated membranes and stop diarrhea with a cup or two of this astringent and anti-inflammatory tea.

Yield: 1 cup | **Prep time:** 5 minutes, plus 10 to 15 minutes to infuse

INGREDIENTS: 1 cup of water, 1 to 2 teaspoons of dried and chopped agrimony (aerial parts), 1 teaspoon of dried and chopped echinacea (optional), and raw honey

SUPPLIES: A teakettle or pot for heating water, an empty tea bag or infuser, and a teacup

1. Heat the water in the teakettle.
2. While the water is heating, fill the tea bag with agrimony (and echinacea, if using).
3. Carefully pour the water into the teacup and then add the tea bag. Allow this to infuse for 10 to 15 minutes.
4. Add a small amount of raw honey to taste and let it cool enough to drink.
5. Drink 1 cup as needed, and do not exceed 3 cups daily.

Boneset and Echinacea Antiviral Tea

Has a viral fever got you down? Try this potent antiviral tea blend to feel better faster.

Yield: 1 cup | **Prep time:** 5 minutes, plus 10 to 15 minutes to infuse

INGREDIENTS: 1 cup of water, 1 teaspoon of dried and chopped boneset (aerial parts), 1 teaspoon of dried and chopped echinacea, and raw honey

SUPPLIES: A teakettle or pot for heating water, an empty tea bag or infuser, and a teacup

1. Heat the water in the teakettle.
2. While the water is heating, fill the tea bag with boneset and echinacea, if using.
3. Carefully pour the water into the teacup, then add the tea bag. Allow this to infuse for 10 to 15 minutes.
4. Add a small amount of raw honey to taste and let it cool enough to drink.
5. Drink 1 to 2 cups a day, preferably at the onset of a viral infection.

Clear Skin Burdock Tea

For skin so healthy it glows, try drinking
a cup of burdock tea daily.

Yield: 1 cup | **Prep time:** 5 minutes,
plus 10 to 15 minutes to infuse

INGREDIENTS: 1 cup of water, 2 teaspoons of dried and chopped
burdock root, and raw honey

SUPPLIES: A teakettle or pot for heating water, an empty tea bag
or infuser, and a teacup

1. Heat the water in the teakettle.
2. While the water is heating, fill the tea bag with burdock root.
3. Carefully pour the water into the teacup and add the tea bag. Allow this to infuse for 10 to 15 minutes.
4. Add a small amount of raw honey to taste and let it cool enough to drink.

Calendula Skin-Healing Oil

Apply this versatile oil infusion to wounds, rashes, bumps, bruises, and any other skin conditions for healing, inflammation reduction, and elimination of redness and irritation.

Yield: 4 ounces | **Prep time:** 5 minutes, plus 8 to 10 hours to infuse

INGREDIENTS: Enough calendula flowers to fill a 4- to 6-ounce jar and enough carrier oil (jojoba is my favorite for this recipe) to completely cover the plant material

SUPPLIES: A 4- to-6-ounce jar for infusion, a medium-size pan, a strainer or cloth, a small bowl, a small funnel, and at least four 1-ounce dropper bottles

1. Fill a 4- to 6-ounce jar with dried calendula flowers.
2. Completely cover the flowers with the carrier oil.
3. Place the jar in a pan of hot water on the "warm" setting of your stove. If you don't have a warm setting, place it on a burner on low. Fill the water in the pan high enough that it rises above most of the contents of the jar, but not so high that it might spill into the oil and plant material.
4. Let this infuse for 8 to 12 hours. I like to let mine go even longer to better infuse the plant material into the oil.
5. Pour through a strainer or cloth into a small bowl. I prefer a cloth, because it better allows me to squeeze the remaining oil out of the plant material. Cheesecloth is especially good for this.
6. Using a small funnel, pour the contents of the bowl into the dropper bottles.
7. Massage a small amount into affected areas as needed. Store your oil infusion in a cool, dark place.

Soothing California Poppy Tea

If you or your child is feeling overstimulated and restless, try a cup of this gentle and calming tea.

Yield: 1 cup | **Prep time:** 5 minutes, plus 10 to 15 minutes to infuse

INGREDIENTS: 1 cup of water, 1 to 2 teaspoons of chopped California poppy (aerial parts), and raw honey

SUPPLIES: A teakettle or pot for heating water, an empty tea bag or infuser, and a teacup

1. Heat the water in the teakettle.
2. While the water is heating, fill the tea bag with California poppy.
3. Carefully pour the water into the teacup and add the tea bag. Allow this to infuse for 10 to 15 minutes.
4. Add a small amount of raw honey to taste and let it cool enough to drink.

Tip: For children, try giving them a cup of this tea 2 to 3 hours before bedtime so they don't have to get up in the night to use the bathroom.

Comforting Catnip Compress

Soak a clean cloth in this catnip-infused water and place this on the forehead or neck to bring down a fever. You can also apply this compress to other areas of the body for relief from soreness, stiffness, and tired muscles.

Yield: 1 cup | **Prep time:** 10 to 15 minutes, plus time to cool

INGREDIENTS: 2 cups of water and 2 tablespoons of dried and chopped catnip

SUPPLIES: A pot for boiling water, a strainer, a jar or bowl to store the liquid, and a clean cloth to dip in the liquid

1. Bring the water to a boil on the stove and add the catnip.
2. Allow this to boil uncovered until the water is reduced to 1 cup.
3. Remove from the heat and allow this to cool completely before straining it out.
4. Strain the liquid into a jar or bowl and dip a cloth into the jar with the liquid.
5. Allow the cloth to fully soak up the liquid. Wring it out a bit before applying it to the skin.
6. Apply as needed to the neck or head to bring down a fever.

Tip: For a soothing muscle compress, you don't have to allow the liquid to cool. You can dip the cloth in the liquid when it is still warm (just make sure it isn't too hot to apply to skin).

Pain and Circulation Cayenne Salve

Massage this soother into swollen joints, painful areas (do not get into open wounds), or areas that need increased blood circulation.

Yield: Around 8 ounces | **Prep time:** 25 minutes, plus several hours to cool and harden

INGREDIENTS: 1 ounce of beeswax pellets, about 8 ounces of carrier oil, 1 tablespoon of cayenne powder (you can use the powder you find in the spice aisle of your supermarket), and 5 to 10 drops of ginger essential oil (optional, but ginger is also anti-inflammatory and analgesic, and complements the cayenne well)

SUPPLIES: 1 double boiler and 4 (2-ounce) tins with lids

1. Place the double boiler on the stove, fill the bottom halfway to three-quarters with water, and turn the heat to low.

2. Place the beeswax pellets in the top of the double boiler and allow these to melt completely.

3. When the pellets have melted, add the carrier oil and then the cayenne powder, and stir continually for 15 minutes.

4. Remove the double boiler from the heat and add the ginger essential oil (if using). Stir again for 2 to 3 minutes until the oil is blended well.

5. Carefully pour this into tins. Allow this preparation several hours to cool and harden. It can take a while for the salve to reach the right consistency. You can speed up this process by placing the tins in the refrigerator for a few hours. Store in a cool, dry place.

Reduce-the-Redness Chamomile Skin Toner

Use a cotton ball to apply this toner to the face to promote healthy, balanced skin.

Yield: 2 ounces | **Prep time:** 20 minutes, plus up to 6 hours to infuse

INGREDIENTS: 1 ounce of distilled water, 1 tablespoon of dried chamomile flowers, and 1 ounce of food-grade aloe vera juice

SUPPLIES: A small pot for boiling water, a jar, a 2-ounce bottle for storing the toner, a small funnel, a strainer, and a cotton ball

1. Bring the distilled water just to a boil.

2. As the water is heating, fill a mason jar with chamomile flowers.

3. When the water has started boiling, carefully pour it into the jar with the flowers, and allow this to infuse for up to 6 hours.

4. Using the funnel, fill the storage bottle with 1 ounce of aloe vera juice.

5. Strain out the chamomile infusion and, using the funnel, pour the liquid into the bottle with the aloe vera juice. Shake everything well to blend it together.

6. Place some liquid on a cotton ball and apply to clean facial skin up to twice daily.

7. Between uses, store in the refrigerator, where it should last up to 2 weeks.

Cooling Chickweed Salve

This salve is just what skin needs to heal, hydrate, and bring out a healthy, soft glow.

Yield: Around 8 ounces | **Prep time:** 10 minutes, plus 4 to 6 weeks to infuse and several hours to cool and harden

INGREDIENTS: Enough wilted or dried chickweed to fill an 8-ounce glass jar, about 8 ounces of carrier oil, and 1 ounce of beeswax pellets

SUPPLIES: An 8-ounce mason jar, a strainer or straining cloth, a small bowl (it should be able to hold 8 ounces of oil), a double boiler, and 4 tins with lids (2-ounce size)

1. To make this salve, you have to make a plant-infused oil first. To do this, fill an 8-ounce mason jar with wilted or dried chickweed.

2. Completely cover the plant material in the jar with the carrier oil.

3. Place a lid on the jar and allow this to sit and infuse for 4 to 6 weeks. Shake your jar daily to further promote infusion.

4. After 4 to 6 weeks, strain out the oil into a small bowl.

5. Place the double boiler on the stove, fill the bottom halfway to three-quarters with water, and turn the heat to low.

6. Place the beeswax pellets in the top of the double boiler and allow these to melt completely.

7. When the pellets have melted, carefully pour the strained oil into the beeswax and blend everything together well.

8. Remove the double boiler from the heat and carefully pour the mixture into the tins. Allow this several hours to cool and harden. It can take a while for the salve to reach the right consistency. You can speed up this process by placing the tins in the refrigerator for a few hours.

9. Apply a liberal amount of this salve as needed to rashes and other skin irritations. Store in a cool, dry place.

Lymph Support Cleavers Tincture

Use this tincture in the spring to help your lymphatic system recover from a long winter.

Yield: 4 ounces | **Prep time:** 10 minutes, plus 4 to 6 weeks to infuse

INGREDIENTS: Enough chopped fresh cleavers to fill a 4-ounce glass jar and about 4 ounces of at least 80 proof alcohol

SUPPLIES: A 4-ounce jar (a little bigger than this is fine), a strainer, another jar for after straining, a small funnel, and 2 (2-ounce) dropper bottles

1. Fill one of the jars with cleavers.

2. Completely cover the cleavers in at least 80 proof alcohol.

3. Place a lid on the jar and allow to infuse for 4 to 6 weeks. Store the jar in a cool, dark place.

4. Shake the jar daily to further promote infusion.

5. Strain out the liquid into another jar. Using a small funnel, carefully pour the preparation into 2 labeled dropper bottles.

6. Take 1 dropperful up to 3 times daily in the spring months. Store in a cool, dry place.

"Bone Knit" Comfrey Salve

Comfrey salve can be massaged into swollen, painful areas of the body to promote healing by reducing swelling and even bruising.

Yield: Around 8 ounces | **Prep time:** 10 minutes, plus 4 to 6 weeks to infuse and several hours to cool and harden

INGREDIENTS: Enough dried and chopped comfrey leaves to fill an 8-ounce glass jar, about 8 ounces of a carrier oil, and 1 ounce of beeswax pellets

SUPPLIES: An 8-ounce mason jar, a strainer or straining cloth, a small bowl (it should be able to hold 8 ounces of oil), a double boiler, and 4 tins with lids (2-ounce size)

1. Fill an 8-ounce mason jar with dried and chopped comfrey leaves.

2. Completely cover the plant material in the jar with a carrier oil.

3. Place a lid on the jar and allow this to sit and infuse for 4 to 6 weeks.

4. Shake your jar daily to further promote infusion.

5. Strain the oil into the small bowl.

6. Place the double boiler on the stove, fill the bottom halfway to three-quarters with water, and turn the heat to low.

7. Place the beeswax pellets in the top of the double boiler, and allow these to melt completely.

8. When the pellets have melted, carefully pour the strained oil in the bowl into the beeswax and blend everything together well.

continues >>

"Bone Knit" Comfrey Salve *continued*

9. Remove the double boiler from the heat and carefully pour the preparation into the tins. Allow several hours to cool and harden. It can take a while for the salve to reach the right consistency. You can speed up this process by placing the tins in the refrigerator for a few hours.

10. Apply a liberal amount of this salve as needed to bumps, bruises, fractures, sprains, and other areas of trauma. Do not ingest or apply to open wounds. Store in a cool, dry place.

Cottonwood Balm of Gilead

Balm of Gilead can be massaged into swollen, painful areas of the body to promote healing by reducing swelling and even bruising.

Yield: Around 8 ounces | **Prep time:** 10 minutes, plus 4 to 6 weeks to infuse, 8 hours for jar to warm, and several hours for the mixture to cool and harden

INGREDIENTS: Enough cottonwood buds to fill an 8-ounce jar, about 8 ounces of carrier oil, and 1 ounce of beeswax pellets

SUPPLIES: An 8-ounce mason jar, medium-size pan, a strainer or straining cloth, a small bowl (it should be able to hold 8 ounces of oil), a double boiler, and 4 tins with lids (2-ounce size)

1. Fill an 8-ounce mason jar with cottonwood buds.

2. Completely cover the plant material in the jar with a carrier oil.

3. Place a lid on the jar and allow this to sit and infuse for 4 to 6 weeks. Shake your jar daily to further promote infusion.

4. Before straining, place the jar in a pan of hot water on the "warm" setting of your stove. If you don't have a warm setting, place it on a burner on low. Fill the water in the pan high enough that it rises above most of the contents of the jar, but not so high that it might spill into the oil and plant material.

5. Strain the oil into a small bowl.

6. Place the double boiler on the stove, fill the bottom halfway to three-quarters with water, and turn the heat to low.

continues >>

Cottonwood Balm of Gilead *continued*

7. Place the beeswax pellets in the top of the double boiler and allow these to melt completely.

8. When the pellets have melted, carefully pour the strained oil into the beeswax and blend everything together well.

9. Remove the double boiler from the heat and carefully pour it into tins. Allow several hours to cool and harden. You can speed up this process by placing the tins in the refrigerator for a few hours.

10. Apply a liberal amount of this salve as needed to arthritic joints, bumps, bruises, fractures, sprains, and other painful or inflamed areas. Do not apply to open wounds. Store in a cool, dry place.

Dandelion Tonic Tea

Dandelion root tea is the perfect tonic
to support healthier skin and skin tone.

Yield: 1 cup | **Prep time:** 5 minutes,
plus 10 to 15 minutes to infuse

INGREDIENTS: 1 cup of water, 2 to 3 teaspoons of dried and
chopped dandelion root, and raw honey

SUPPLIES: A teakettle or pot for heating water, an empty tea bag
or infuser, and a teacup

1. Heat the water in the teakettle.
2. While the water is heating, fill the tea bag with
   dandelion root.
3. Carefully pour the water into the teacup and add the tea
   bag. Allow this to infuse for 10 to 15 minutes.
4. Add a small amount of raw honey to taste and let it cool
   enough to drink.
5. Drink 1 to 2 cups daily.

Echinacea Sore Throat Gargle

This is a powerful remedy for killing bacteria in the throat responsible for sore, inflamed tonsils and adenoids.

Yield: 1 quart | **Prep time:** 10 minutes,
plus 8 to 10 hours to infuse

INGREDIENTS: A quart of water and ½ cup of chopped purple coneflower (aerial parts and roots)

SUPPLIES: Pot for boiling water, 2 (1-quart) jars, and a strainer or straining cloth

1. Start by bringing the water to a boil on the stove.

2. While the water is heating, fill one of the mason jars with the chopped purple coneflower parts.

3. When the water comes to a boil, carefully pour this into one of the mason jars until the water reaches the top.

4. Place a lid on the jar and allow this to sit and infuse for 8 to 10 hours (it helps to start this process at night before bed to infuse while you sleep).

5. Strain out the water through a strainer or straining cloth, and store it in another quart mason jar in the refrigerator.

6. To use, gargle around 20 to 30 milliliters for up to a minute before spitting it out. Do this every few hours until symptoms are gone. Use within 1 week.

Storage tip: For a longer shelf life, pour the infusion into ice cube molds and freeze overnight. Then place the cubes into a labeled freezer bag and thaw as needed. This will help your infusion last up to 1 year.

Amber's "Famous" Elderberry Glycerite

This potent elderberry remedy uses non-GMO, food-grade vegetable glycerin as the solvent for the extract. I prefer fresh-harvested berries when making this.

Yield: About ½ quart | **Prep time:** 3 hours 15 minutes, plus 4 weeks to infuse

INGREDIENTS: 1 quart of freshly harvested elderberries (if using dried, you will need to add a bit of water to the recipe), a few sticks of Ceylon cinnamon, small, freshly sliced ginger root (optional), and enough vegetable glycerin to cover the berries in a quart jar

SUPPLIES: 1 (1-quart) glass jar, a large pot for boiling, cheesecloth, a large bowl, a funnel, and 4 (4-ounce) bottles for storage (I prefer tinted glass bottles for this recipe)

1. Fill a quart jar with elderberries (if using dried, add $\frac{1}{2}$ cup of water to the jar afterward). Add a few sticks of Ceylon cinnamon and some small slices of ginger (if using).

2. Completely cover the berries in non-GMO, food-grade vegetable glycerin. This will take some time, because vegetable glycerin is thick and viscous. Pour small amounts at a time until it covers the berries.

3. Place a lid on the jar and shake it as best you can. It will shake better as the days go by and the berries begin to infuse their juice and medicinal compounds into the glycerin.

4. Store in a cool, dry place for 4 weeks. Make sure to shake daily.

continues >>

Amber's "Famous" Elderberry Glycerite *continued*

5. Dump the contents of the jar—berries, cinnamon, ginger (if using), and glycerin—into a pot.

6. Turn up the heat to medium and slowly bring the mixture to a boil.

7. Let boil for 3 minutes before turning down the heat and allowing it to simmer for up to 3 hours. The heat is great for further infusing the berries into the vegetable glycerin.

8. Turn off the heat. When cool enough to touch, strain the contents of the pot through a cheesecloth and into a large bowl. Squeeze the berries in the cheesecloth to get all their medicinal goodness. I ask my husband to do this because he has a very powerful grip and can get a lot of liquid out of the spent berries.

9. Use a funnel to pour this liquid into the bottles for storage. Placing in the refrigerator will extend the shelf life up to 6 months or more.

10. We take 5 (for kids) to 10 (for adults) milliliters up to 3 times a day at the first sign of illness. The medicine cups that come with some over-the-counter medicines are good for measuring the doses.

Bye-Bye Bloating Fennel Tea

Drink a cup of this tea as needed to experience quick relief from bloating, gas, and other digestive issues.

Yield: 1 cup | **Prep time:** 5 minutes, plus 10 to 15 minutes to infuse

INGREDIENTS: 1 cup of water, 2 teaspoons of fennel seeds, and raw honey

SUPPLIES: A teakettle or pot for heating water, an empty tea bag or infuser, and a teacup

1. Heat the water in the teakettle.
2. While the water is heating, fill the tea bag with fennel seeds.
3. Carefully pour the water into the teacup and add the tea bag. Allow this to infuse for 10 to 15 minutes.
4. Add a small amount of raw honey to taste and let cool enough to drink.
5. Drink 1 cup as needed for bloating, gas, indigestion, constipation, and other digestive issues.

Goldenrod Urinary Support Tea

Drink 1 to 3 cups of this tea daily at the
first sign of a UTI, or 1 cup daily to help prevent
an infection (if you are prone to them).

Yield: 1 cup | **Prep time:** 5 minutes,
plus 10 to 15 minutes to infuse

INGREDIENTS: 1 cup of water, 2 to 3 teaspoons of dried and
chopped goldenrod (aerial parts), and raw honey

SUPPLIES: A teakettle or pot for heating water, an empty tea bag
or infuser, and a teacup

1. Heat the water in the teakettle.

2. While the water is heating, fill the tea bag with goldenrod.

3. Carefully pour the water into the teacup and add the tea
   bag. Allow this to infuse for 10 to 15 minutes.

4. Add a small amount of raw honey to taste and let it cool
   enough to drink. (Don't add too much, as sugar can feed
   an infection or make it worse).

5. Drink 1 to 3 cups throughout the day at the first sign of an
   infection. You can also drink a cup a day for maintenance
   if you are prone to UTIs.

Tranquility Hops Tea

If you need a gentle sedative to quiet the mind and body, help you sleep at night, or prevent night sweats, try a cup of this tea in the evening before bed.

Yield: 1 cup | **Prep time:** 5 minutes, plus 10 to 15 minutes to infuse

INGREDIENTS: 1 cup of water, 2 to 3 teaspoons of dried hops flowers, and raw honey

SUPPLIES: A teakettle or pot for heating water, an empty tea bag or infuser, and a teacup

1. Heat the water in the teakettle.
2. While the water is heating, fill the tea bag with hops.
3. Carefully pour the water into the teacup and add the tea bag. Allow this to infuse for 10 to 15 minutes.
4. Add a small amount of raw honey to taste and let it cool enough to drink.
5. Drink 1 cup an hour or two before bed for help with sleep or as needed to calm the nerves.

Honeysuckle Antiviral Tincture

Feel a virus coming on? When you detect the telltale signs of an approaching viral infection, start taking this tincture right away.

Yield: 4 ounces | **Prep time:** 10 minutes, plus 4 to 6 weeks to infuse

INGREDIENTS: Enough Japanese honeysuckle vine (I harvest when it is in full bloom) to fill a 4-ounce jar and about 4 ounces of at least 80 proof alcohol

SUPPLIES: 2 (4-ounce) glass jars (a little bigger is fine), a strainer, a small funnel, and 2 (2-ounce) dropper bottles

1. Fill one of the jars with chopped honeysuckle vine.

2. Completely cover the plant material in at least 80 proof alcohol.

3. Place a lid on the jar and allow this to infuse for 4 to 6 weeks. Store the jar in a cool, dark place.

4. Shake the jar daily to further promote infusion.

5. Strain the liquid into another jar. Using a small funnel, carefully pour the preparation into the labeled dropper bottles and label them.

6. Take 1 dropperful every 3 hours throughout the day at the first sign of illness. Store in a cool, dry place.

Winter Blues Juniper Bath Soak

Soak in this uplifting bath blend to melt away stiffness, pain, and inflammation in the muscles while also treating your skin with an infusion of antioxidants to experience healthier, glowing skin.

Yield: 1 cup | **Prep time:** 15 minutes, plus 4 to 6 weeks to infuse

INGREDIENTS: Enough juniper berries to fill a 2-ounce jar, about ¼ cup of a carrier oil (my favorite for this recipe is jojoba oil), and 1 cup of Epsom salts

SUPPLIES: A 2-ounce jar, a strainer, a small bowl for straining the oil into, and a bowl for blending the ingredients together

1. Fill a 2-ounce mason jar with juniper berries.

2. Completely cover the plant material in the jar with a carrier oil. I like jojoba oil, but you can use anything you think will work for your skin.

3. Place a lid on the jar and allow this to sit and infuse for 4 to 6 weeks.

4. Shake your jar daily to further promote infusion.

5. Strain out the oil into a small bowl. This juniper berry oil infusion can be used on its own to massage into sore muscles, if you don't feel like making a bath soak.

6. In another bowl, add 1 cup of Epsom salts.

7. Blend the strained oil with the Epsom salts. Keep stirring until everything is blended thoroughly.

8. Feel free to add more Epsom salts until you reach a consistency you like. Sometimes I add a tablespoon of crumbled juniper berries to the blend as well. This is completely optional.

9. Add this preparation to a warm bath, and soak as long as you like for relief and skin health.

Skin-Soothing Lavender and Aloe Spray

Use this soothing spray on a sunburn, heat rash, or any other red and inflamed skin area to decrease inflammation, redness, and help promote healing. Best of all, the spray bottle requires no contact with the skin, so there's no flinching in pain when the remedy is applied.

Yield: 8 ounces | **Prep time:** 20 minutes, plus time to cool

INGREDIENTS: About 4 ounces of distilled water, 3 teaspoons of dried lavendar buds, and 4 ounces of food-grade aloe vera juice

SUPPLIES: Small pot for heating water, a strainer, a small bowl, a small funnel, and an 8-ounce spray bottle

1. Heat the water on the stove and add the lavender buds. Allow this to come to a boil and then let it simmer for 10 to 15 minutes.

2. Remove the pot from heat and let it cool before straining it out.

3. Strain the lavender water into a small bowl and then add the aloe vera juice. Blend these together well.

4. Place a funnel on the spray bottle and pour the contents of the bowl into the bottle.

5. Apply this spray as often as needed to burns and other skin issues for quick relief and healing.

6. Between uses, store the spray bottle in the refrigerator, where it should last for up to 3 weeks. Always discard water-based remedies if you notice any mold in the liquid (even if it occurs before the 2- to 3-week expiration).

Lemon Balm Ice Pops

These lemon balm ice pops don't just cool you off on a hot summer's day. They also help calm the nerves and soothe the body and mind, and they're safe to eat for children or adults.

Yield: 12 ounces | **Prep time:** 15 to 20 minutes, plus overnight to freeze

INGREDIENTS: 1½ cups of water, ½ cup of chopped lemon balm (fresh or dried), and raw honey

SUPPLIES: A pot for boiling water, a strainer, a jar to strain the liquid into, and ice pop molds

1. Bring the water to a boil on the stove.

2. When the water comes to a boil, carefully add the lemon balm and allow this to simmer over medium heat for 10 minutes.

3. Strain out the liquid into a jar.

4. Add raw honey to taste (start with a tablespoon and go from there).

5. Gently stir in the honey until it dissolves in the warm water.

6. Carefully pour the liquid into ice pop molds and freeze overnight.

7. Enjoy as needed for a sweet and beneficial summer treat.

8. Feel free to get creative! Add fruit, edible flowers, juice, or anything else to make something unique to you and your needs.

Tip: Add a tablespoon or two of chopped catnip to the lemon balm in the pot as you boil. This helps make a doubly soothing and calming treat that children and adults can safely enjoy.

Coating Marshmallow Infusion

Drink a cup of this gentle infusion to coat
the stomach, intestines, and urinary tract with a soothing,
natural gel that comes from marshmallow root.

Yield: 1 quart | **Prep time:** 5 to 10 minutes,
plus 8 to 10 hours to infuse

INGREDIENTS: 1 quart of water and ½ cup of chopped
marshmallow roots

SUPPLIES: A pot for boiling water, a quart-sized jar, a strainer, and
a sterilized quart mason jar (see page 28) for storage

1. Bring a quart of water to a boil on the stove.

2. While waiting for the water to come to a boil, fill a quart jar with marshmallow roots.

3. When the water has come to a boil, gently pour it into the mason jar with the plant material.

4. Place a lid on the jar and allow this to sit and infuse for 8 to 10 hours.

5. Strain out the liquid when it cools and store it in a sterilized glass quart jar in the refrigerator.

6. Drink 1 to 2 cups of this infusion daily or as needed to manage digestive or urinary pain and spasms.

Mimosa Happiness in a Bottle

Take 1 to 2 dropperfuls of this synergistic tincture if you're in need of some emotional healing and restoration.

Yield: 4 ounces | **Prep time:** 10 minutes, plus 4 to 6 weeks to infuse

INGREDIENTS: Enough mimosa flowers, twigs, and inner bark to fill a 4-ounce jar and about 4 ounces of at least 80 proof alcohol

SUPPLIES: A 4-ounce glass jar (a little bigger is fine), a strainer, another jar for after straining, a small funnel, and 2 (2-ounce) dropper bottles

1. Fill a jar with mimosa pieces.
2. Completely cover the plant material in at least 80 proof alcohol.
3. Place a lid on the jar and allow this to infuse for 4 to 6 weeks. Store the jar in a cool, dark place.
4. Shake the jar daily to further promote infusion.
5. Strain the liquid into another jar. Using a small funnel, carefully pour it into the labeled dropper bottles.
6. Take 1 to 2 dropperfuls as needed. Store in a cool, dry place.

Quick Relief Motherwort Remedy

This tincture recipe works quickly for my clients, and I have had people rave about how effective it was when they wanted immediate relief for anxiety and stress.

Yield: 4 ounces | **Prep time:** 10 minutes, plus 4 to 6 weeks to infuse

INGREDIENTS: Enough motherwort to fill a 4-ounce jar and about 4 ounces of at least 80 proof alcohol

SUPPLIES: A 4-ounce glass jar (a little bigger is fine), a strainer, another jar for after straining, a small funnel, and 2 (2-ounce) dropper bottles

1. Fill one of the jars with chopped motherwort.
2. Completely cover the plant material in at least 80 proof alcohol.
3. Place a lid on the jar and allow this to infuse for 4 to 6 weeks. Store the jar in a cool, dark place.
4. Shake the jar daily to further promote infusion.
5. Strain out the liquid into another jar. Using a small funnel, carefully pour the liquid into the labeled dropper bottles.
6. Take 1 dropperful as needed during times of stress and anxiety. Hold the tincture under your tongue up to 30 seconds before swallowing it. If it's too strong for your taste, dilute it in a glass of water before taking it. Store in a cool, dry place.

Respiratory Support
Mullein Tincture

This tincture can be taken to break up congestion and open the airways for those who are having issues with bronchitis, respiratory viruses, and allergies.

Yield: 4 ounces | **Prep time:** 10 minutes, plus 4 to 6 weeks to infuse

INGREDIENTS: Enough mullein leaves (chopped) to fill a 4-ounce jar and about 4 ounces of at least 80 proof alcohol

SUPPLIES: 2 (4-ounce) glass jars (a little bigger is fine), a strainer or straining cloth, a small funnel, and 2 (2-ounce) dropper bottles

1. Fill a 4-ounce jar with chopped mullein leaves. They can be either fresh or dried.

2. Completely cover the plant material in at least 80 proof alcohol and place the lid on the jar. Store it in a cool, dark place for 4 to 6 weeks.

3. Shake the jar daily to further promote infusion.

4. Strain out the liquid through a strainer or straining cloth and into the other jar.

5. Placing a small funnel in the dropper bottles, carefully pour the liquid from the jar into the dropper bottles.

6. Take 2 dropperfuls every 2 to 3 hours as needed for respiratory support. Store in a cool, dry place.

Antimicrobial Oregano Oil Infusion

This antimicrobial oil infusion is awesome for massaging around the ears (not in the ear canal) to help with ear infections. It can also be applied to fungal skin issues and skin infections.

Yield: 4 ounces | **Prep time:** 5 minutes, plus 8 to 12 hours to infuse

INGREDIENTS: Enough dried and chopped oregano to fill a 4- to 6-ounce jar and enough carrier oil (olive oil is my favorite for this recipe) to completely cover the plant material

SUPPLIES: A 4- to 6-ounce jar for infusion, a medium-size pan, a strainer or cloth, a small bowl, a small funnel, and at least 4 (1-ounce) dropper bottles

1. Fill a 4- to 6-ounce jar with dried and chopped oregano.
2. Completely cover the plant material with the carrier oil.
3. Place the jar in a pan of hot water on the "warm" setting of your stove. If you don't have a warm setting, place it on a burner on low. Fill the water in the pan high enough that it rises above most of the contents of the jar, but not so high that it might spill into the oil and oregano.
4. Let this infuse for 8 to 12 hours. I like to let mine go even longer to better infuse the plant material into the oil.

5. Strain out the plant material through a strainer or cloth into a small bowl. I prefer a cloth because it allows me to squeeze the remaining oil out of the plant material better.

6. Use a small funnel to pour the contents of the bowl into the dropper bottles.

7. Massage a small amount into affected areas as needed.

8. Store your oil infusion in a cool, dark place.

Mental Exhaustion Passionflower Tincture

Adults should take 2 dropperfuls of this tincture as needed for stress and anxiety.

Yield: 4 ounces | **Prep time:** 10 minutes, plus 4 to 6 weeks to infuse

INGREDIENTS: Enough passionflower (chopped aerial parts—make sure to include plenty of flowers) to fill a 4-ounce jar and about 4 ounces of at least 80 proof alcohol

SUPPLIES: A 4-ounce glass jar (a little bigger is fine), a strainer, another jar for after straining, a small funnel, and 2 (2-ounce) dropper bottles

1. Fill one of the jars with chopped passionflower vine and flowers.
2. Completely cover the plant material in at least 80 proof alcohol.
3. Place a lid on the jar and allow to infuse for 4 to 6 weeks. Store the jar in a cool, dark place.
4. Shake the jar daily to further promote infusion.
5. Strain out the liquid into another jar. Using a small funnel, carefully pour the liquid into the labeled dropper bottles.
6. Take 2 dropperfuls as needed. Store in a cool, dry place.

Digestive Support Peppermint Infusion

If you suffer from irritable bowel syndrome, nausea, digestive upset, bloating, gas, or intestinal spasms, this infusion can help bring much-needed relief.

Yield: 1 quart | **Prep time:** 10 minutes, plus 8 to 10 hours to infuse

INGREDIENTS: 1 quart of water and 1 ounce of peppermint leaves

SUPPLIES: A pot to boil water, a quart mason jar with a lid, a strainer, and a sterilized quart jar (see page 28) to store the infusion

1. Bring a quart of water in a pot to a boil on the stove.

2. While waiting for the water to come to a boil, fill a quart jar with 1 ounce of peppermint leaves (double if using fresh leaves).

3. When the water has come to a boil, gently pour it into the mason jar with the plant material.

4. Place a lid on the jar and allow to sit and infuse for 8 to 10 hours.

5. Strain out the liquid when it cools, and store it in a sterile glass jar in the refrigerator.

6. Drink 2 to 3 cups of this infusion daily or as needed.

Pine Pitch Salve

Massage this powerful salve into your chest as needed when you feel congested to help open airways and promote respiratory health during times of sickness.

Yield: Yield will vary depending on how much sap you are able to collect. A good rule of thumb is 2 parts olive oil to 1 part pine pitch and 1 part beeswax to 4 parts combined pitch and oil. | **Prep time:** 1 to several days (including pine sap collection)

INGREDIENTS: 1 part pine sap, 2 parts extra-virgin olive oil, and 1 part beeswax pellets to 4 parts combined oil and pitch

SUPPLIES: A double boiler, a strainer (optional), and a jar for storing your salve

1. Melt the sap and olive oil using a double boiler filled halfway to three-quarters with water using low heat. It may take a second for the sap to fully melt, so be patient! Never try to melt pine sap under a direct flame, as it can be flammable.

2. If you want, you can strain the oil and sap blend at this time, but this is optional. Sometimes a few pieces of wood, etc. get in the sap as you are collecting it. If this bothers you, simply strain it through a filter at this time before returning it to the double boiler.

3. Once everything has liquified, add the beeswax and stir until it melts into the oil and sap blend.

4. Once the beeswax has melted, pour this into a jar (or jars, depending on how much you make) to cool.

5. Place a lid on the jar when it has cooled and store it in a cool, dark place for use as needed.

Tip: I love adding 5 to 10 drops of pine, cedarwood, or fir needle essential oils to this recipe after the beeswax has melted and the double boiler has been removed from heat. This creates an even more powerful and aromatic salve.

Calming Pineapple Weed Tea

Enjoy a cup of this tasty tea when you
need to relax the body and mind.

Yield: 1 cup | **Prep time:** 5 minutes,
plus 10 to 15 minutes to infuse

INGREDIENTS: 1 cup of water, 1 to 2 teaspoons of chopped pineapple weed (aerial parts), and raw honey (optional)

SUPPLIES: A teakettle or pot for heating water, an empty tea bag or infuser, and a teacup

1. Heat the water in the teakettle.

2. While waiting for the water to heat, fill an infuser or empty tea bag with 1 to 2 teaspoons of chopped pineapple weed (you can use fresh or dried).

3. When the water has sufficiently heated, carefully pour it into a teacup.

4. Place the tea bag into the water and allow this to infuse for 10 to 15 minutes. Add the honey to taste (if using).

5. Enjoy 1 to 2 cups as needed for stress, anxiety, insomnia, or muscle spasms.

Quick Plantain Poultice

Harvest a leaf as needed to apply to wounds, contusions, rashes, splinters, bug bites, stings, and any other skin irritation for quick relief.

Yield: Around 1 teaspoon | **Prep time:** 1 minute

INGREDIENTS: 1 plantain leaf and a teaspoon or less of distilled water, or tap water if that's all you have

SUPPLIES: A mortar and pestle

1. Harvest a plantain leaf and wash it thoroughly.

2. Crush up the leaf into pieces and place these inside a mortar and pestle.

3. Mash up the leaf pieces until you have a pliable ball of mush that can be applied to a wound, etc. You can add tiny amounts of water until this consistency is reached.

4. Apply this to the affected area and cover it with a bandage. Reapply as needed.

Tip: Old-timers used to chew the leaf and then spit it out and apply it to the affected area. Since that isn't the most sanitary thing to do, I suggest mashing a leaf in between your fingers and applying this to a wound in a pinch. (This is especially helpful if you don't have a mortar and pestle.)

Allergy-Busting Purple Deadnettle Tincture

The quercetin in purple deadnettle helps suppress histamine response in the body, lowering inflammation and other allergy symptoms. Take 2 dropperfuls of this tincture as needed for allergy relief.

Yield: 4 ounces | **Prep time:** 10 minutes, plus 4 to 6 weeks to infuse

INGREDIENTS: Enough purple deadnettle (aerial parts) to fill a 4-ounce jar and about 4 ounces of at least 80 proof alcohol

SUPPLIES: 2 (4-ounce) glass jars (a little bigger is fine), a strainer, a small funnel, and 2 (2-ounce) dropper bottles

1. Fill one of the jars with chopped purple deadnettle.
2. Completely cover the plant material in at least 80 proof alcohol.
3. Place a lid on the jar and allow to infuse for 4 to 6 weeks. Store in a cool, dark place.
4. Shake the jar daily to further promote infusion.
5. Strain out the liquid into another jar. Using a small funnel, carefully pour the liquid into the labeled dropper bottles.
6. Take 2 dropperfuls every 3 to 4 hours as needed for allergy relief. Store in a cool, dry place.

Red Clover Hormonal Balance Infusion

Drink 2 to 3 cups of this infusion daily to help balance hormones and support cardiovascular health.

Yield: 1 quart | **Prep time:** 10 minutes, plus 8 to 10 hours to infuse

INGREDIENTS: 1 quart of water and 1 ounce of dried red clover flowers

SUPPLIES: A pot to boil water, a quart mason jar with a lid, a strainer, and a sterile jar (see page 28) to store the infusion

1. Bring a quart of water in a pot to a boil on the stove.
2. While waiting for the water to come to a boil, fill a quart jar with one ounce of dried red clover flowers.
3. When the water has come to a boil, gently pour it into the mason jar with the plant material.
4. Place a lid on the jar and allow this to sit and infuse for 8 to 10 hours.
5. Strain out the liquid when it cools and store it in a sterile glass jar in the refrigerator.
6. Drink 2 to 3 cups of this infusion daily or as needed.

Uterine-Nourishing Red Raspberry Tea

Drink 1 to 2 cups of this tea daily or as needed to encourage toning of the uterus and reduce menstrual discomfort.

Yield: 1 cup | **Prep time:** 5 minutes, plus 10 minutes to infuse

INGREDIENTS: 1 cup of water, 1 to 2 teaspoons of dried and chopped red raspberry leaves, and raw honey (optional)

SUPPLIES: Teakettle or pot for heating water, an empty tea bag, and a teacup

1. Heat 1 cup of water on the stove. It doesn't have to be boiling, just steaming.

2. While you are waiting for your water to heat, fill an empty tea bag with red raspberry leaves.

3. When the water has heated, pour it into your teacup and place the tea bag into the cup.

4. Allow this to infuse for 10 minutes.

5. Let it cool enough to safely drink, and add some raw honey if desired.

Rosemary Hair Thickening and Growth Mask

Apply this nourishing mask to your hair once or twice weekly for best results. I also add 2 teaspoons to my shampoo and conditioner (and shake it really well before use) to get even more benefits from this oil infusion.

Yield: 4 ounces | **Prep time:** 5 to 10 minutes, plus 8 to 12 hours to infuse

INGREDIENTS: Enough dried and chopped rosemary (aerial parts) to fill a 4-ounce glass jar, about 3 ounces of jojoba oil, and 1 ounce of castor oil

SUPPLIES: A 4-ounce glass jar, a small-size pan, a strainer or cloth, a small bowl, and another 4-ounce glass jar for storage

1. Fill one of the jars with rosemary and then completely cover it with the jojoba and castor oils (no plant material should be sticking out).

2. Place the jar in a pan of hot water on the "warm" setting of your stove. If you don't have a warm setting, place it on a burner on low. Fill the water in the pan high enough that it rises above most of the contents of the jar, but not so high that it might spill into the oil and plant material.

3. Let this infuse for 8 to 12 hours. I like to let mine go even longer to better infuse the plant material into the oil.

4. Strain out the plant material through a strainer or cloth into a small bowl. I prefer a cloth, like cheesecloth, because it allows me to squeeze the remaining oil out of the plant material better.

continues >>

Rosemary Hair Thickening and Growth Mask

continued

5. Store your strained oil in a jar and keep it in a cool, dark place between uses.

6. Massage a liberal amount of this rosemary-infused oil blend into the scalp and work your way down the shaft of hair. Leave it in for 20 minutes before rinsing with warm water, then wash as usual.

Cold Sore–Busting Self-Heal Lip Balm

This remedy can help eliminate cold sores while also leaving your lips silky smooth.

Yield: Around 3 ounces | **Prep time:** 10 minutes, plus 4 to 6 weeks to infuse and several hours to cool and harden

INGREDIENTS: 2 to 3 tablespoons of dried and chopped self-heal (aerial parts), 2 tablespoons plus 2 teaspoons of a carrier oil, 2 tablespoons of beeswax pellets

SUPPLIES: A small, sterile glass jar (see page 28) for infusing the plant in oil, a strainer or cloth, a double boiler, a small funnel, 4 to 6 empty lip balm tubes

1. Fill a sterile glass jar with the plant material and then completely cover it in a carrier oil.

2. Let this sit (with the lid on the jar) for 4 to 6 weeks.

3. Shake the jar daily to further promote infusion.

4. Strain out the oil into a small bowl (it helps to do this through a cloth so you can squeeze the plant material to get all the oil out) and set aside.

5. Place the double boiler on the stove, fill the bottom halfway to three-quarters with water, and turn the heat to low. Add the beeswax to the top and allow it to melt thoroughly.

6. Once the beeswax has melted, add the plant-infused oil by carefully pouring it from the bowl into the double boiler.

7. Blend everything together well. Using a small funnel, carefully pour the mixture into the lip balm tubes.

continues >>

Cold Sore–Busting Self-Heal Lip Balm *continued*

8. Allow the tubes to sit for several hours to cool and harden. Placing them in the refrigerator can speed up this process.

9. Apply this every few hours at the first sign of a cold sore. Store in a cool, dry place.

Tip: Lemon balm is another great plant for viral lesions. Adding 5 to 10 drops of lemon balm essential oil to this salve when it's still in liquid form (before pouring the salve into containers) is a great way to give maximum potency to this recipe. Blend it in well before pouring into containers.

Unwind and Relax
Skullcap Tincture

If you're feeling stressed and need to unwind, try
2 dropperfuls of skullcap tincture to calm the nerves.

Yield: 4 ounces | **Prep time:** 10 minutes,
plus 4 to 6 weeks to infuse

INGREDIENTS: Enough skullcap (chopped aerial parts) to fill a
4-ounce jar and about 4 ounces of at least 80 proof alcohol

SUPPLIES: A 4-ounce glass jar (a little bigger is fine), a strainer,
another jar for after straining, a small funnel, and
2 (2-ounce) dropper bottles

1. Fill a jar with chopped skullcap.

2. Completely cover the plant material in at least
   80 proof alcohol.

3. Place a lid on the jar and allow this to infuse for 4 to
   6 weeks. Store the jar in a cool, dark place.

4. Shake the jar daily to further promote infusion.

5. Strain the liquid into another jar. Using a small funnel,
   carefully pour this preparation into the labeled
   dropper bottles.

6. Take 2 dropperfuls as needed to unwind. Store in a cool,
   dry place.

St. John's Wort Bottle of Sunshine

If you need a pick-me-up, St. John's wort tincture has got your back. Its gentle nervine properties can help you see the bright side and calm your frazzled nerves.

Yield: 6 ounces | **Prep time:** 5 to 10 minutes, plus 4 to 6 weeks to infuse

INGREDIENTS: Enough St. John's wort flowers to fill a 6-ounce jar (you can include a few leaves as well) and about 6 ounces of at least 80 proof alcohol

SUPPLIES: A 6-ounce glass jar for infusion, a strainer, a small funnel, 3 (2-ounce) tinted dropper bottles

1. Fill a 6-ounce jar with St. John's wort flowers (and a few leaves if you wish).

2. Completely cover the plant material in at least 80 proof alcohol.

3. Place a lid on the jar and store it in a cool, dark place for 4 to 6 weeks.

4. Shake the jar daily to further promote infusion.

5. Strain out the liquid and, using a small funnel, pour it into the labeled dropper bottles.

6. Take 1 to 2 dropperfuls up to three times daily for SAD, anxiety, stress, nerve pain, or mild to moderate depression. Store in a cool, dry place.

Nourishing Nettle Broth

This nutritious broth is perfect for sipping before and after surgery, childbirth, or sickness to replenish vitamins, minerals (like iron), and other nutrients the body needs to recover. Feel free to be creative with this recipe and add other ingredients as you see fit. You can use vegetable broth if you prefer.

Yield: Around one quart | **Prep time:** 25 minutes

INGREDIENTS: 1 quart of organic chicken or turkey broth, 1 cup of dried stinging nettle, 2 garlic cloves, ⅓ medium-size onion (sliced), and any other herbs you wish to add (such as rosemary, oregano, and thyme)

SUPPLIES: A stock pot

1. In a stockpot, combine the broth, stinging nettle, garlic, onion, and herbs.

2. Gradually increase the heat from low to medium.

3. Allow the contents of the pot to come to a boil, then reduce the heat and let this simmer, covered, for 15 to 20 minutes.

4. Remove the pot from the heat and allow it to cool a bit before enjoying. Drink 1 to 2 cups daily as needed for recovery.

Sweet Gum Influenza Tincture

For best results, use this tincture alongside honeysuckle or elderberry at the first indication of viral illness. This combination works especially well against influenza.

Yield: 4 ounces | **Prep time:** 10 minutes, plus 4 to 6 weeks to infuse

INGREDIENTS: Enough finely chopped green (unripe) sweet gum seedpods to fill a 4-ounce jar and about 4 ounces of at least 80 proof alcohol

SUPPLIES: A 4-ounce glass jar (a little bigger is fine), a strainer, another jar for after straining, a small funnel, and 2 (2-ounce) dropper bottles

1. Fill a jar with chopped sweet gum seedpods.

2. Completely cover the plant material in at least 80 proof alcohol.

3. Place a lid on the jar and allow this to infuse for 4 to 6 weeks. Store the jar in a cool, dark place.

4. Shake the jar daily to further promote infusion.

5. Strain out the liquid into another jar and then, using a small funnel, carefully pour the preparation into the labeled dropper bottles.

6. Take 1 dropperful every 3 hours throughout the day at the first indication of viral illness. Store in a cool, dry place.

Sweet Wormwood Antiviral Tincture

Adults should take 2 dropperfuls of this tincture up to three times daily at the first sign of illness. This recipe shouldn't be taken by children or someone who's pregnant.

Yield: 4 ounces | **Prep time:** 10 minutes, plus 4 to 6 weeks to infuse

INGREDIENTS: Enough sweet wormwood (chopped aerial parts) to fill a 4-ounce jar and about 4 ounces of at least 80 proof alcohol

SUPPLIES: A 4-ounce glass jar (a little bigger is fine), a strainer, another jar for after straining, a small funnel, and 2 (2-ounce) dropper bottles

1. Fill one of the jars with the sweet wormwood parts.
2. Completely cover the plant material in at least 80 proof alcohol.
3. Place a lid on the jar and allow this to infuse for 4 to 6 weeks. Store the jar in a cool, dark place.
4. Shake the jar daily to further promote infusion.
5. Strain out the liquid into another jar. Using a small funnel, carefully pour the preparation into the labeled dropper bottles.
6. Take 1 to 2 dropperfuls up to three times daily. Store in a cool, dry place.

Sandman Valerian Tea

Drink this tea 1 hour to 30 minutes before you go to bed to get a more restful night's sleep.

Yield: 1 cup | **Prep time:** 5 minutes, plus 10 to 15 minutes to infuse

INGREDIENTS: 1 cup of water, 1 to 2 teaspoons of chopped valerian root, and raw honey (optional)

SUPPLIES: A teakettle or pot for heating water, an empty tea bag or infuser, and a teacup

1. Heat the water in the teakettle.

2. While the water is heating, fill the tea bag with valerian root.

3. Carefully pour the water into the teacup and add the tea bag. Allow this to infuse for 10 to 15 minutes.

4. Add a small amount of raw honey to taste (if using) and let cool enough to drink.

Soothing Violet Infusion

When allergies, a raw throat, sinus issues, or annoying coughs are making you miserable, try a cup of this infusion to ease irritation and quell the cough. Add a bit of raw honey for an even more powerful and tasty remedy.

Yield: 1 quart | **Prep time:** 5 to 10 minutes, plus 8 to 10 hours to infuse

INGREDIENTS: A quart of water, and ½ cup each of violet flowers and leaves (fresh is best)

SUPPLIES: A pot for boiling water, a quart jar, a strainer, and a sterile quart jar (see page 28) for storage

1. Bring a quart of water in a pot to a boil on the stove.

2. While waiting for the water to come to a boil, fill a quart jar with the violet flowers and leaves.

3. When the water has come to a boil, gently pour it into the mason jar with the plant material.

4. Place a lid on the jar and allow the remedy to sit and infuse for 8 to 10 hours.

5. Strain out the liquid when it cools, and store it in a sterile glass jar in the refrigerator.

6. Drink 1 to 2 cups of this infusion as needed.

Headache White Willow Tincture

Take this tincture when you feel a headache coming on for fast relief. It's also great for reducing a fever and treating pain and inflammation in other areas of the body.

Yield: 4 ounces | **Prep time:** 10 minutes, plus 4 to 6 weeks to infuse

INGREDIENTS: Enough white willow bark to fill a 4-ounce jar and about 4 ounces of at least 80 proof alcohol

SUPPLIES: A 4-ounce glass jar (a little bigger is fine), a strainer, another jar for after straining, a small funnel, and 2 (2-ounce) dropper bottles

1. Fill one of the jars with shavings of white willow bark.
2. Completely cover the plant material in at least 80 proof alcohol.
3. Place a lid on the jar and allow this to infuse for 4 to 6 weeks. Store the jar in a cool, dark place.
4. Shake the jar daily to further promote infusion.
5. Strain out the liquid into another jar. Using a small funnel, carefully pour the liquid into the labeled dropper bottles.
6. Take 1 to 3 dropperfuls every 4 to 6 hours as needed for pain, inflammation, and fevers. Store in a cool, dry place.

Wild Bergamot Oxymel

Take a 1-ounce shot of this invigorating and stimulating oxymel to soothe symptoms of a viral infection. Its antimicrobial properties also make it helpful for throat infections. The measurements in the ingredients section are estimates, not exact amounts. When filling the jar, I usually add 1 to 2 parts apple cider vinegar and 2 to 3 parts honey. Too much apple cider vinegar can make the taste quite strong.

Yield: Around 4 ounces | **Prep time:** 10 minutes, plus 4 to 6 weeks to infuse

INGREDIENTS: Enough wild bergamot flowers (and a few leaves if you prefer) to fill a 4-ounce jar, about 1½ ounces of raw, organic apple cider vinegar, and about 2½ ounces of raw honey

SUPPLIES: A 4-ounce jar (a little bigger is fine), a strainer or straining cloth, and another 4-ounce jar for storage

1. Fill a jar with wild bergamot flowers and leaves. I prefer using fresh plant material, but if you are using dried, you don't have to fill the jar all the way to the top—just halfway.

2. Add the apple cider vinegar and honey. Make sure the plant material is completely covered.

3. Place a lid on the jar and store it in a cool, dark place for 4 to 6 weeks.

4. Shake the jar daily to further promote infusion.

5. Strain out the contents of the jar into another jar for storage. (Be prepared for it to be sticky and messy.)

6. Store your oxymel in a cool, dark place, and take an ounce shot as needed for viruses or infections.

Wild Rose Beauty Serum

Apply a small amount of this serum to the face, neck, and chest daily. Use a carrier oil that works best for your particular skin needs. I prefer a light oil like sweet almond or grapeseed oil, because they do not clog pores.

Yield: 4 ounces | **Prep time:** 5 to 10 minutes, plus 8 to 12 hours to infuse

INGREDIENTS: An equal blend of dried rose hips and petals (enough to fill a 4- to 6-ounce jar) and enough carrier oil (sweet almond or grapeseed oil are my favorites for this recipe) to completely cover the plant material

SUPPLIES: A 4- to 6-ounce jar for infusion, a medium-size pan, a strainer or cloth, a small bowl, a small funnel, and at least 4 (1-ounce) dropper bottles

1. Fill a 4- to 6-ounce jar with rose petals and hips.

2. Completely cover the plant material with a carrier oil.

3. Place the jar in a pan of hot water on the "warm" setting of your stove. If you don't have a warm setting, place it on a burner on low. Fill the water in the pan high enough that it rises above most of the contents of the jar, but not so high that it might spill into the oil and plant material.

4. Let this infuse for 8 to 12 hours. I like to let mine go even longer to better infuse the plant material into the oil.

5. Strain out the plant material through a strainer or cloth into a small bowl. I prefer a cloth like cheesecloth, because it allows me to squeeze more of the remaining oil out of the plant material.

6. Use a small funnel to pour the oil into the dropper bottles.

7. Massage a small amount into the skin of your face, neck, and chest daily.

8. Store your oil infusion in a cool, dark place.

Toning Witch Hazel Facial Spray

Mist your face, neck, and chest with this soothing spray in the morning (and evening if you have extra-oily skin) for clearer skin and an improved skin tone.

Yield: Around 18 ounces | **Prep time:** 20 minutes, plus time to cool

INGREDIENTS: ½ pound of witch hazel bark, leaves, and flowers, enough distilled water to cover the plant material in a pot on the stove, and about 8 ounces of at least 80 proof organic vodka (optional for longer shelf life)

SUPPLIES: A pot for boiling on the stove, a strainer, a bowl, a funnel, and a large spray bottle for storing the toner

1. Pour the witch hazel and distilled water into a pot on the stove.

2. Bring this to a boil and then turn down the heat and allow it to simmer, covered, for 15 minutes.

3. Remove the pot from heat and keep it covered until it has cooled.

4. Strain out the liquid into a bowl and then add the vodka (again, this is optional, but it helps extend the shelf life from 1 week to 1 to 2 years). Alcohol is more drying, but for those with oily skin, that can be helpful. If you have sensitive skin, leave the alcohol out.

5. Using a funnel, pour the mixture into the spray bottle. Store it in the refrigerator for a cooling facial treatment. An alcohol-free version of this will last in the refrigerator 1 week. With the alcohol, it will remain potent for a year or more.

Yarrow Styptic Powder

Treat cuts, lacerations, and other wounds with this powder to stop bleeding, kill germs, and promote swift healing. Keep it in your natural first aid kit to have ready when you need it.

Yield: 1 ounce | Prep time: 15 to 20 minutes

INGREDIENTS: 1 ounce (or more if you desire) of dried yarrow leaves

SUPPLIES: A mortar and pestle and a small, sterile glass jar (see page 28) with a lid for storage

1. Add the dried plant material to the mortar and pestle and grind to a powder consistency. This can take some time, so turn on your favorite show or podcast as you grind away!

2. Once you have ground the leaves into powder, store the powder in a sterile glass jar with a lid and keep it in a cool, dry place.

3. Apply the powder straight to cuts and leave it there for up to 15 minutes (or longer if you desire).

4. Once the bleeding has stopped, remove the powder by gently washing it off with soap and water. Any extra powder can be stored in a cool, dry place.

Digestive Health Yellow Dock Infusion

If you suffer from constipation, an upset stomach, bloating, or anemia, then an infusion of yellow dock may provide relief while helping cleanse the body.

Yield: 1 quart | **Prep time:** 5 to 10 minutes, plus 8 to 10 hours to infuse

INGREDIENTS: A quart of water and 1 cup of chopped yellow dock root (and some leaves if you wish)

SUPPLIES: A pot for boiling water, a quart jar, a strainer, and a sterilized quart jar (see page 28) for storage

1. Bring a quart of water to a boil in a pot on the stove.
2. While waiting for the water to come to a boil, fill one of the quart jars with yellow dock.
3. When the water has come to a boil, gently pour it into the jar with the plant material.
4. Place a lid on the jar and allow this to sit and infuse for 8 to 10 hours.
5. Strain out the liquid when it cools, and store in a sterilized glass jar in the refrigerator.
6. Drink 1 to 2 cups of this infusion daily or as needed for digestive issues. It lasts up to 1 week if refrigerated.

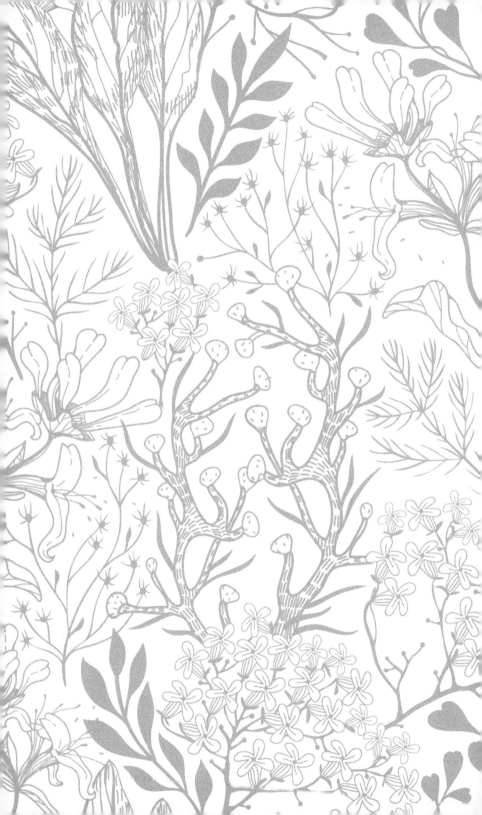

Resources

American Herbalist's Guild (AHG)

americanherbalistsguild.com

National Institutes of Health

nih.gov

Science Direct Journals

sciencedirect.com | Science, health, and medical journals and full-text articles and books.

United Plant Savers

unitedplantsavers.org

References

Catanzaro, Michele, et al. "Immunomodulators Inspired by Nature: A Review on Curcumin and Echinacea." *Molecules* 23, no. 11 (2018): 2778. doi.org/10.3390/molecules23112778.

Chan, Yuk-Shing, et al. "A Review of the Pharmacological Effects of *Arctium Lappa* (Burdock)." *Inflammopharmacology* 19 (2011): 245–254. doi.org/10.1007/s10787-010-0062-4.

Ho, Giang Thanh, et al. "Elderberry and Elderflower Extracts, Phenolic Compounds, and Metabolites and Their Effect on Complement, RAW 264.7 Macrophages and Dendritic Cells." *International Journal of Molecular Sciences* 18, no. 3 (2017): 584. doi.org/10.3390/ijms18030584.

Orege, Joshua Iseoluwa, et al. "*Artemisia* and *Artemisia*-Based Products for COVID-19 Management: Current State and Future Perspective." *Advances in Traditional Medicine* (2012): 1–12. doi.org/10.1007/s13596-021-00576-5.

Panahi, Yunes, et al. "Rosemary Oil vs. Minoxidil 2% for the Treatment of Androgenetic Alopecia: A Randomized Comparative Trial." *Skinmed* 13, no. 1 (January–February 2015): 15–21. PMID: 25842469.

Petrovska Biljana Bauer. "Historical Review of Medicinal Plants Usage." *Pharmacognosy Reviews* 6, no. 11 (May 2012): 1–5. doi.org/10.4103/0973-7847.95849.

Index

About the Author

 AMBER ROBINSON, PhD, is an American Herbalists Guild registered herbalist, National Association for Holistic Aromatherapy level 2 professional aromatherapist, author, and instructor at The Bitter Herb Academy, an online school she founded in 2016. Dr. Robinson spends her days wildcrafting and growing plant medicine on her 80-acre homestead in the Missouri Ozarks.